# BABY NA

*FANTASTIC AND UNIQUE NAMES FOR GIRLS AND BOYS*

By

*RUSTY COVE-SMITH*

**ISBN 9781790581030**

Thank you for supporting our work.

https://gimbooks.info/team/rusty-cove-smith/

# WHY YOU SHOULD READ THIS BOOK

If you're searching for unique and amazing baby names, you've chosen the right book!

Nowadays fewer parents are picking popular names for their children, but going for uncommon ones instead, that's why I decided to write this book.

A name is the first thing we learn about a person. It's how they're presented to the world. It's the defining declaration a parent makes when labeling their children.

Every one-of-a-kind baby should have his/her **Unique baby name** as an individual; each baby is special!

**Enjoy finding unique names for baby on our baby names lists.**

# TABLE OF CONTENTS

"BEFORE THE INTERNET, NO ONE REALIZED HOW POPULAR CERTAIN NAMES WERE, BUT NOW THE INFORMATION IS OUT THERE."

CLEVELAND EVANS,

FORMER PRESIDENT OF THE AMERICAN NAME SOCIETY

# CHAPTER 1. UNIQUE BABY NAMES A TO F

## LETTER A:

▶♂**Abdiel:** In the Bible, Abdiel was the name of the ancient prophet who could withstand Satan. This name means 'servant of God.' (Chronicles 5:15)

**Pronunciation:** [Ăb'dĭel] or AB-dee-el

*For 2017, the number of births with name Abdiel is 373, which represents 0.019 percent of total male births in 2017.*

**Related to:** Abdal, Abdel, Abdi, Abdullah, Avdiel.

## ▶♀**Aerin (or Aeryn):** Pronunciation: AY-rin

This name derived from the Gaelic Érinn, the dative case of Érie, which is the Irish name for Ireland. Though this name is popular in the UK and the U.S., it is not normally bestowed as a given name in Ireland.

Aerin is also considered of Hebrew origin meaning Enlightened, being related to the male name Aaron

*For 2017, the number of births with name Aerin is 37, which represents 0.0022 percent of total female births in 2017.*

**Related Names:** Aeron, Erin, Aaron.

►♂**Aidan (also Aiden or Aedan)** are the main anglicization of the Irish male given name Aodhán and the Scottish Gaelic given name Aodhàn.

**Pronunciation:** /ˈeɪdən/

In Gaelic, the meaning of the name Aidan is Little fire, ardent. (born of fire/the fiery one/little fiery one).

**Related Names:** Aodhán Hayden, Ayden, Aden, Aydan, and Aydin.

*For 2017, the number of births with name Aidan is 1718, which represents 0.088 percent of total male births in 2017.*

►♀**Aislinn:** derived of Aisling an Irish name, meaning 'dream' or vision, or day-dream.

**Related to:** Ashlynn or Ashlyn and the Anglicized name: Esther.

*For 2016, the number of births with name Aislinn is 277, which represents 0.014 percent of total female births in 2016.*

**Pronunciation:** ASH-lin or AYZ-lin.

►♀**Aitana:** is the name of a Spanish mountain in the Costa Blanca Area (Alicante), was used for the first time by the Spanish poet Rafael Alberti. But it was popularized via Aitana Sanchez Gijan, the famous Spanish actress (Alberti's goddaughter).

**Pronunciation:** "eye ta na" or "ie-TA-na"

*For 2017, the number of births with name Aitana is 422, which represents 0.023 percent of total female births in 2017.*

▶♀**Aliana and Alianna** are both 21st-century American name inventions most likely inspired by Alice/Allie and Ana. Alianna could also be considered a slight variation of Elianna (like Aileen vs. Eileen). Elianna is derivative of the Hebrew Eliyanah which means "God has answered me" or the "Lord has responded."

**Similar names:** Arianna, Adrianna and Audrianna.

**Pronounced:** Al-lee-ah-na, Al-lee-an-na

*For 2017, the number of births with name Alianna is 240, which represents 0.014 percent of total female births in 2017.*

▶♀**Alaia:** Alternately from the Basque, meaning "joyful or happy."

**Pronunciation:** ah-LIY-ə.

*For 2017, the number of births with name Alaia is 460, which represents 0.025 percent of total female births in 2017.*

It may be related as well to Aaliyah is a variation of the name Aliyah, which means "rising" in Hebrew and "exalted or lofty" in Arabic. Other variations include Alia, Aleah, Aleia, Alya and Aliyya.

▶♂**Alasdair:** Scottish name, the Gaelic form of Alexander - meaning "defender of mankind" or "the one who repels men."

**Related to:** Alexander, Alistair, Alastair, Alaster, Alastor.

*For 2017, the number of births with name Alasdair is 21, which represents 0.0011 percent of total male births in 2017.*

**Pronunciation:** 'A'-les-dare

▶♀**Alessandra:** Derived from the Greek Alexandros, a male compound name composed of the elements alexein (to defend, to help) and Andros (man), see Alasdair.

**Pronunciation:** ah-leh-SAHN-drə.

**Similar names:** Alexandra, Alessa, Lessa, Alexi.

*For 2017, the number of births with name Alessandra is 1034, which represents 0.055 percent of total female births in 2017.*

▶♀**Allegra:** Derived from the Latin *"allegro"* (cheerful, happy. lively). In Music, "allegro" which is used to instruct the musician to perform with an upbeat and lively sound.

**Pronunciation:** ə-LEG-rə (English), ahl-LE-grah (Italian).

**Related names:** Allegria, Allegrina, Aggie.

*For 2017, the number of births with name Allegra is 71, which represents 0.0041 percent of total female births in 2017.*

▶♀**Amaia or Amaya:** From the word Amainera that means "the end" in Basque. Amaia is also the name of a mountain and a village in the Basque region of Spain. Other origins: Japanese for "night rain" and in Aymara Culture in South America for "Beloved Daughter" or "long wished Daughter."

**Pronunciation:** ah-MIY-ə

*For 2017, the number of births with name Amaya is 1709, which represents 0.091 percent of total female births in 2017 and Amaia is not in the top 1000 names for any year of birth beginning with 1900.*

▶♂**Andre:** From the Greek word Andreios, which means manly or brave.

**Pronunciation:** AHN-dray.

**Similar names:** Andreas, Andrew, Anders, Ander, Deanre.

*For 2017, the number of births with name Andre is 1356, which represents 0.069 percent of total male births in 2017.*

▶♀**Anja:** Finnish variation of Anna which is is a Latinate variant of the French Anne, a cognate of the Hebrew Hannah or "chaanach" (gracious, full of grace).

**Pronunciation:** AHN-yə.

**Related to:** Anna, Hannah, Annika, Anya, Hana.

*For 2017, the number of births with name Anja is 63, which represents 0.0037 percent of total female births in 2017.*

▶♂**Antwan:** From the Latin *"Antonius,"* an old Etruscan and Roman word of unknown etymology. "Priceless" and "of inestimable worth" are popular folk definitions of the name. It Is the African American version of Antoine or Anthony.

**Pronounced:** an-TWAHN

**Similar names:** Anton, Antonio, Anthony, and Antoine.

*For 2017, the number of births with name Antwan is 105, which represents 0.0057 percent of total male births in 2017.*

▶♂**Apollo:** Apollo is a Greek name, derived from the verb *"apollymi"* meaning to destroy or perhaps from the Greek word Apollōn. In Greek mythology by the handsome son of Zeus and Leto and twin brother of the goddess Artemis. Apollo, one of the twelve major deities, was the god of music, poetry, prophecy, and medicine. Later he also became the god of the sun and light.

**Pronunciation:** ah-PAH-loh or ə-PAW-lo.

*For 2017, the number of births with name Apollo is 525, which represents 0.027 percent of total male births in 2017.*

**Similar names:** Apollon.

▶ ♀**Arden:** From an English surname, originally taken from various place names, which were derived from a Celtic word "Ardu" meaning "high" or "high land." Arden is a unisex name, used as a boy name and a girl name.

**Pronunciation:** AHR-dən

*For 2017, the number of births with name Arden is 225, which represents 0.013 percent of total female births in 2017.*

▶ ♂**Arlo:** is a short name, probably originated as a nickname for Carlos, Carlo or Marlow. Perhaps inspired by the fictional place name Arlo Hill from the poem 'The Faerie Queene' (1590) by Edmund Spenser. Aherlow is a Gaelic word that means "between two highlands." Also, is the Basque word for "area." It is believed that may be derived from the Anglo-Saxon *here* or 'army, fortified, troops.

**Pronunciation:** AHR-loh.

*For 2017, the number of births in the U.S. with name Arlo is 1084, which represents 0.055 percent of total male births in 2017.*

► ♂**Aramis:** French origin, first coined by Alexandre Dumas in his novel The Three Musketeers as the name of one of the protagonists in that book (whose surname was derived from the French village of Aramits).

**Pronunciation:** A RA mis

*For 2017, the number of births with name Aramis is 55, which represents 0.003 percent of total male births in 2017.*

► ♀**Ariadne:** Ariadne is the lesser-known form of the name Ariana. Besides, it's also the name of the Cretan goddess of fertility. Ariadne was the daughter of King Minos. She fell in love with Theseus and helped him to escape the Labyrinth and the Minotaur but was later abandoned by him. Eventually, she married the god Dionysus.

**Pronounced:** ar-ee-AD-nee.

**Related to:** Ariadna, Ariana, Arianna, Arianne.

*For 2017, the number of births with name Ariadne is 353, which represents 0.019 percent of total female births in 2017.*

▶♀**Astrid:** Modern form of ÁSTRÍÐR, Derived from the Old Norse elements áss "god" and fríðr "beautiful, beloved."

**Related to:** Astride, Asta and Sassa.

*For 2017, the number of births with name Astrid is 399, which represents 0.021 percent of total female births in 2017.*

**Pronunciation:** ASS-trid

▶♀**Athena:** A cognate of the Greek Athēnē, an ancient name of unknown etymology borne in Greek mythology by the goddess of wisdom, skill, and warfare. Athena is the patron goddess of the city of Athens in Greece. It is likely that her name is derived from that of the city, not vice versa.

**Pronunciation:** ah-THEE-nə

**Similar to:** Athina and Athene

*For 2017, the number of births with name Athena is 2365, which represents 0.126 percent of total female births in 2017.*

▶♂**Atlas:** Possibly means "not enduring" from Greek "tlao" and the negative prefix "a." In Greek mythology, he was a Titan punished by Zeus by being forced to support the heavens on his shoulders.

**Pronunciation:** AT-lass.

*For 2017, the number of births with name Atlas is 1034, which represents 0.053 percent of total male births in 2017.*

▶♀**Audrina:** comes from Audrey (with the popular name suffix -ina) which means *'noble strength'*.

Pronounced; aw--DREE-nah, aw-DREE-na

**Other Forms:** Audreena, Audrena

*For 2017, the number of births with name Audrina is 318, which represents 0.017 percent of total female births in 2017.*

▶♀**Augusta:** Feminine form of AUGUSTUS. Which Means "great" or "venerable," derived from Latin augere "to increase."

**Pronounced:** ow-GUWS-ta

**Variant:** Auguste

*For 2017, the number of births with name Athena is 66 which represents 0.0039 percent of total female births in 2017.*

# LETTER B:

▶ ♀♂**Bailey:** from the Old French/English word baili (manager), which is derived from bailiff / bailiff (an officer of justice or a warrant officer).

**Pronunciation:** BAY-lee

**Similar to:** Bailee, Baylee.

*For 2017, the number of births with name Bailey is 2420, which represents 0.129 percent of total female births in 2017. For 2017, the number of births with name Bailey is 141, which represents 0.0077 percent of total male births in 2017.*

▶ ♂**Bannon:** English surname used as a (mostly) male name. Anglicized form of the Old Gaelic Irish surname O' Banain, which means "son of the fair-haired one."

**Pronunciation:** BA-nən or BANN-uhn

*For 2017, the number of births with name Bannon is 10, which means its located in the 7500th place for male names in 2017.*

▶ ♂**Barnabas:** a name is borne in the Bible by the Christian apostle and missionary companion of Paul. The name is derived from the Aramaic barnebhū'āh meaning son of exhortation or encouragement (Acts 4:36).

**Similar to:** Barnaby

**Pronounced as** BAR nah bus

*For 2017, the number of births in the U.S. with the name Barnabas is 24, which means its located in the 4194th place for male names in 2017.*

▶♂**Bartholomew:** From the word "Bartholomaios" a Greek form of the Aramaic name meaning "son of Talmai." Talmai is an Aramaic name meaning "hill, mound, furrows." The name is borne in the Bible by one of the Twelve Apostles of Christ.

**Short form or nickname:** Bart.

**Pronunciation:** bahr-THAHL-ǝ-myoo

*For 2017, the number of births in the U.S. with the name Bartholomew is 21, which means its located in the 4568th    place for male names in 2017.*

▶♀**Bee:** Short form of Beatrix, Probably from Viatrix, a feminine form of the Late Latin name Viator which meant "voyager, traveler." It was a common name amongst early Christians, and the spelling was altered by association with Latin *beatus meaning* "blessed, happy."

**Similar to:** Beatrice, Beatrix, Bea, Beatriz.

*For 2017, the number of births with name Bee is less than 5.*

▶ ♀**Belinda:** Of uncertain origin and meaning, it has been suggested that the name is of Germanic origin, possibly a variant of Betlindis, which is thought to mean "snake" or "serpent." Or maybe related to Italian/Spanish word Bella which means Beautiful.

**Pronounced:** bə-LIN-də

**Related /short name:** Bindy

*For 2017, the number of births with name Belinda is 169, which represents 0.009 percent of total female births in 2017.*

▶ ♀**Bella:** Derived from the Latin bella (beautiful). Short form of Isabella or any other name ending in bella.

**Similar names:**  Belle, Isabelle, Isabella.

**Pronunciation:** BEHL-ə

*For 2017, the number of births with name Bella is 4611, which represents 0.246 percent of total female births in 2017.*

▶ ♀**Bette:** Diminutive of Elizabeth, derived from the Hebrew elīsheba' (God is my oath).

**Similar names:** Betty

Pronounced: Like Bet or Be-tty

*For 2017, the number of births with name Bee is less than 5.*

▶♀**Bianca:** Derived from the Italian word "Bianca," meaning white.

**Pronunciation:** bee-AHN-kə.

**Similar to:** Blanche

*For 2017, the number of births with name Bianca is 827, which represents 0.044 percent of total female births in 2017.*

▶♂**Booker:** name related to the occupational surname meaning "maker of books."

**Pronounced:** BUWK-ər

*For 2017, the number of births with name Booker is 83, which represents 0.0045 percent of total male births in 2017.*

▶♂**Boyd:** From a Scottish surname which was possibly derived from the name of the island of Bute.

**Pronunciation:** BOYD

*For 2017, the number of births with name Boyd is 122, which represents 0.0067 percent of total male births in 2017.*

►♀**Brigitte:** Anglicized form of the Gaelic Bríghid, which is believed to be derived from brígh (strength).

**Pronunciation:** bri-ZHEET, bri-GEE-tə

**Similar names:** Bridget

*For 2017, the number of births with name Brigitte is 64, which represents 0.0037 percent of total female births in 2017.*

# LETTER C:

▶♀**Cadimhe or Caoimhe:** From the Gaelic, meaning "Gentle, kind, Beautiful."

**Pronunciation:** Kee+va or key+va but Irish usual pronounce it like quee+va.

*For 2017, the number of female births with name Cadimhe is 13.*

▶♀**Cara:** Derived from the Latin *"cara"* (beloved) or the Irish Gaelic cara (friend). Alternatively, Cara is used as a short form of Caroline and Charlotte.

**Pronunciation:** KAH-rə, KAYR-ə

For 2017, the number of births with name Cara is 317, which represents 0.017 percent of total female births in 2017.

▶♀**Carine:** French form of Carina. Derived from the Latin *carina* (keel of a ship). Carina is the name of a southern constellation which contains the star Canopus, the second-brightest star in the heavens.

**Pronunciation:** kah-REE-ne

*For 2017, the number of births in the U.S. with name Carine is less than 5.*

▶♂**Caspar:** From Casper, the Dutch form of Gaspar, which, along with Balthasar and Melchior, was assigned to the Three Wise Men who brought gifts to the Christ Child. The names are not found in the Bible and are thought to have been assigned in the 11th century. Of uncertain etymology, Caspar might be derived from the Persian genashber (treasure master), which is in keeping with his role of the bringer of precious gifts.

**Related to:** Gaspar, Casper, Jasper.

**Pronounced:** KAHS-pər.

*For 2017, the number of births with name Caspar is less than 20.*

▶♂**Cedric:** An invention of Sir Walter Scott (1771 - 1832) for the character Cedric the Saxon in *"Ivanhoe"* (1819). He is believed to have based the name on *Cerdic,* a name of uncertain etymology borne by the traditional founder of the West Saxon kingdom.

**Pronunciation:** SEHD-rik or SED-r!k.

*For 2017, the number of births with name Cedric is 207, which represents 0.011 percent of total male births in 2017.*

▶♀**Chanel:** From the French surname meaning "pipe, channel." It has been used as an American given name since the 1970s, influenced by the Chanel brand name.

**Pronunciation:** shə-NEHL

**Related names:** Channa, Shanelle

*For 2017, the number of births with name Chanel is 390, which represents 0.023 percent of total female births in 2017.*

▶♀**Christy:** Diminutive of Christine, as a male name is the diminutive of CHRISTOPHER.

**Pronounced:** KRIS-tee

*For 2017, the number of female births with name Christy is 88, and as a male name less than 5.*

▶♀**Cindy:** Diminutive of Cynthia or Lucinda, Cindy is also bestowed as an independent given name.

**Pronunciation:** SIN-dee

*For 2017, the number of births with name Cindy is 330, which represents 0.013 percent of total female births in 2017.*

*Variants: Cindi, Cyndi, Sindy*

▶♀**Clare:** Medieval English form of Clara, which is derived from the Latin clārus (bright, clear, famous). This is also the name of an Irish county, which was originally named for the Norman invader Richard de Clare, whose surname was derived from the name of an English river.

**Pronunciation:** KLAYR

**Like:** Claire, Clara, Chiara, Clarissa, ...

*For 2017, the number of births with name Clare is 315, which represents 0.017 percent of total female births in 2017.*

▶♀**Claudia:** Feminine form of Claudius, an old Roman family name, which is from claudus (means lame or crippled). It is mentioned briefly in the New Testament.

**Pronounced:** KLAW-dee-ə.

**Related to:** Claud, Claude, Claudette, Claudine, Gladys.

*For 2017, the number of births with name Claudia is 325, which represents 0.017 percent of total female births in 2017.*

▶♀**Cleo:** Short form of Cleopatra, which meant "glory of the father", this was the name of queens of Egypt from the Ptolemaic royal family, including Cleopatra VII, the mistress of both Julius Caesar and Mark Antony. She committed suicide by allowing herself to be bitten by an asp.

**Pronounced:** KLEE-o

*For 2017, the number of births with name Cleo is 157, which represents 0.0088 percent of total female births in 2017 in the U.S.*

▶♀**Coco:** Diminutive of names beginning with Co. However, this was not the case for French fashion designer Coco Chanel (real name Gabrielle), whose nickname came from the name of a song she performed while working as a cabaret singer.

**Pronunciation:** KOH-koh.

*For 2017, the number of births with name Coco is 53, which represents 0.0031 percent of total female births in 2017 in the U.S.*

▶♀**Colette:** Short form of Nicolette which is a diminutive form of Nicole, a feminine form of Nicolas (victory of the people). Saint Colette was a 15th-century French nun who gave her money to the poor.

**Pronunciation:** koh-LEHT

**Related names:** Nicole, Nicolette, Nicky, Nikole

*For 2017, the number of births with name Colette is 578, which represents 0.034 percent of total female births in 2017.*

▶♂**Connell:** From an Irish surname, an Anglicized form of Ó Conaill meaning "descendent of Conall."

**Pronounced:** KAHN-əl

*For 2017, the number of births with name Connell is 19, which represents 0.001 percent of total male births in 2017.*

▶♂**Conner:** Variant of Connor, Anglicized form of the Irish Gaelic Conchobhar, a compound name composed of the elements conn (wisdom, counsel, strength) or con (hound, dog) and cobhair (aid). "High, will, desire" and "hound lover" are other definitions attributed to the name.

**Pronunciation:** KAH-ner

*For 2017, the number of births with name Conner is 1005, which represents 0.051 percent of total male births in 2017.*

▶♀**Constance:** Medieval form of Constantia ("constant, steadfast"), The Normans introduced this name to England (it was the name of a daughter of William the Conqueror).

**Pronounced:** KAHN-stənts or KAHN-stehns.

*For 2017, the number of births with name Constance is 137, which represents 0.008 percent of total female births in 2017.*

▶♀**Consuelo:** Means "consolation" in Spanish. It is taken from the title of the Virgin Mary, Nuestra Señora del Consuelo, meaning "Our Lady of Consolation".

**Pronunciation:** kohn-SWAY-loh

*For 2017, the number of births with name Consuelo is 23, which represents 0.0013 percent of total female births in 2017.*

▶♂**Corban:** Variant of Corbin, a French surname which was derived from corbeau "raven", originally denoting a person who had dark hair.

**Pronounced:** KOR-bin.

*For 2017, the number of births with name Corban is 89, which represents 0.0049 percent of total male births in 2017.*

▶♀**Cordelia:** From Cordeilla, possibly a Celtic name Creiryddlydd (daughter of the sea). The name is borne in Shakespeare's King Lear by Lear's youngest daughter, the only one who was faithful to him.

**Pronunciation:** kohr-DEE-lee-ə, kohr-DEEL-yə.

**Related to:** Cordy / Cordie.

*For 2017, the number of births with name Cordelia is 209, which represents 0.012 percent of total female births in 2017.*

▶♀**Corinne:** French form of Corinna, a Latinized form of the Greek name Κορivvα (Korinna), which was derived from κορη (kore) "maiden."

**Pronounced:** kə-REEN or kə-RIN.

**Variants:** Corine, Corinna, Corrine, Coreen, Corynn, Korrine.

*For 2017, the number of births with name Corinne is 325, which represents 0.017 percent of total female births in 2017.*

▶♂**Crispin:** From the Roman cognomen Crispinus which was derived from the name Crispus ("curly haired"). Saint Crispin was a 3rd-century Roman who was martyred with his twin brother Crispinian in Gaul. They are the patrons of shoemakers.

**Pronunciation:** KRIS-pin

*For 2017, the number of births with name Crispin is 15, which represents 0.0008 percent of total male births in 2017.*

# LETTER D:

▶♂**Daelan:** meaning 'aware.' Used most commonly as a boys' name but can also be used for girls. Its related to Dallan (From the Dale).

**Pronounced as** DEY-LAHN.

**Related names:** Dallan, Dael, Daelin, Daylan...

*For 2017, the number of births with name Daelan is 17, which represents 0.0009 percent of total male births in 2017.*

▶♂**Dale:** From an English surname which originally belonged to a person who lived near a dale or valley.

**Pronunciation:** DAYL

*For 2017, the number of births with name Dale is 150, which represents 0.008 percent of total male births in 2017.*

▶♀**Daphne:** Means "laurel" in Greek. In Greek mythology she was a nymph turned into a laurel tree by her father so that she might escape the pursuit of Apollo. It has been used as a given name in the English-speaking world since the end of the 19th century.

**Pronunciation:** DAF-nee

*For 2017, the number of births with name Daphne is 807, which represents 0.043 percent of total female births in 2017.*

► ♀ **Darcy:** From an English surname which was derived from Norman French d'Arcy, originally denoting one who came from Arcy in France. Darcy was the surname of a character in Jane Austen's novel 'Pride and Prejudice' (1813).

**Pronunciation:** DAHR-see

*For 2017, the number of births with name Darcy is 183, which represents 0.011 percent of total female births in 2017.*

► ♀ **Daria:** Feminine form of Darius, the roman form of the Persian word Dārayavahush (Good possessions), Saint Daria was a 3rd-century Greek woman who was martyred with her husband Chrysanthus.

**Pronounced:** DAHR-ee-ə

*For 2017, the number of births with name Daria is 96, which represents 0.0056 percent of total female births in 2017.*

► ♂ **Daryl:** from Darrel, transferred use of the English surname that originated as the French de Arel (from Airelle, a town in Calvados).

**Pronunciation:** DAR-əl

*For 2017, the number of births with name Daryl is 130, which represents 0.007 percent of total male births in 2017.*

***Similar names:*** *Darrall, Darrel, Darryl, Darylle, Darryll, Daryl.*

▶♀**Deanna:** Originally a variant form of Diana (divine), the name is often used as a feminine form of Dean (a dean).

**Pronunciation:** dee-AN-ə

*For 2017, the number of births with name Deana is 162, which represents 0.009 percent of total female births in 2017.*

▶♂**Devon:** Variant of Devin (from the Gaelic dámh a poet.). It may also be partly inspired by the name of the county of Devon in England.

**Pronunciation:** DEH-vən, də-VAHN

*For 2017, the number of births with name Devon is 416, which represents 0.021 percent of total male births in 2017.*

▶♀**Dinah:** Means "judged" in Hebrew. She is the daughter of Jacob and Leah in the Old Testament.

**Pronunciation:** DIY-nə DYE-nah

*For 2017, the number of births with name Dinah is 51, which represents 0.003 percent of total female births in 2017.*

▶♂**Duff:** Derived from Gaelic dubh meaning "dark."

**Pronounced:** DUF

*For 2017, the number of male births with name Duff is 88, and as a male name less than 5.*

# LETTER E:

▶♂**Eagan:** Transferred from the irish surname, Eagan, (Anglicized) comes from Mac Aodhagáin meaning "son of Aodha" – Aodha meaning "fire" – ultimately in reference to Áed, the ancient Celtic god of fire.

**Pronunciation:** E-gun

*For 2017, the number of births with name Eagan is 15, which represents 0.0008 percent of total male births in 2017.*

▶♀**Edie:** Diminutive of Edith, from the Old English name Eadgyð, derived from the elements ead "rich, blessed" and gyð "war."

**Pronunciation:** EE-dee

*For 2017, the number of births with name Edie is 105, which represents 0.006 percent of total female births in 2017.*

▶♂**Edison:** From an English surname which meant either "son of Eda" or "son of Adam."

**Pronunciation:** EHD-i-sən

*For 2017, the number of births with name Edison is 493, which represents 0.025 percent of total male births in 2017.*

▶♀**Electra:** Latinized form of Greek Ηλεκτρα (Elektra), derived from ηλεκτρον (elektron) meaning "amber." In Greek myth, she was the daughter of Agamemnon and Clytemnestra and the sister of Orestes.

**Other names:** Elettra

*For 2017, the number of births with name Electra is 13, which represents 0.0007 percent of total female births in 2017.*

▶♀**Ekaterina:** the Bulgarian and Macedonian form of Katherine and a variant Russian transcription of Yekaterina (Catherine). Cognate of the Greek Aikaterinē, the root of which is katharos (pure, unsullied).

**Pronunciation:** eh-kah-teh-REE-nə.

*For 2017, the number of births with name Ekaterina is 31, which represents 0.0018 percent of total female births in 2017.*

▶♀♂**Elie:** Short form of Elijah: Derived from the Hebrew 'ēlīyāhū (Jehovah is God). The name was borne by a 9th century B.C. prophet who, after many years of service, was taken up into heaven in a chariot of fire.

**Pronounced:** E-LEE

*For 2017, the number of births with name Elie is 36, which represents 0.002 percent of total male births in 2017. For 2017, the number of births with name Elie is 8, which represents 0.00047 percent of total female births in 2017.*

▶ ♀♂**Elin:** Scandinavian and Welsh form of Helen, English form of the Greek Ἑλένη (Helene), probably from Greek ἑλένη (helene) "torch" or "corposant" or possibly related to σεληνη (selene) "moon." In Greek mythology, Helen was the daughter of Zeus and Leda, whose kidnapping by Paris was the cause of the Trojan War. The name was also borne by the 4th-century Saint Helena, mother of the Roman emperor Constantine.

**Pronunciation:** ee-LYN, EH-lin, EE-ə-lin, EE-ah-lyn.

*For 2017, the number of births with name Elin is 226, which represents 0.013 percent of total female births in 2017, the same year, the number of births with name Elin in a male is 7.*

▶ ♂**Elon:** Means "oak" in Hebrew. Elon was the name of one of the judges of the Israelites in the Old Testament.

**Pronunciation:** EE-lawn

*For 2017, the number of births with name Elon is 188, which represents 0.001 percent of total male births in 2017.*

▶ ♀**Elle:** Diminutive of Eleanor (light, torch, bright) and other names beginning with El. This name can also be given about the French pronoun elle meaning "she."

**Pronunciation:** EHL

*For 2017, the number of births with name Elle is 828, which represents 0.044 percent of total female births in 2017.*

▶ ♂**Ember**: English vernacular form of Jeremiah (the Lord loosens, God will uplift), which dates to the 13th century. In modern times is uses also as sounds like Amber or related to the surname.

**Pronounced:** EM-bər

*For 2017, the number of births with name Ember is 1111, which represents 0.065 percent of total female births in 2017, the same year, the number of births with name Ember in a male is 24.*

▶ ♀**Emmanuelle:** French feminine form of Emmanuel, From the Hebrew name 'Immanu'el meaning "God is with us." This was the foretold name of the Messiah in the Old Testament.

**Pronunciation:** eh-MAN-yoo-EL (English), ay-mahn-WEHL (French)

*For 2017, the number of births with name Emmanuelle is 46, which represents 0.027 percent of total female births in 2017, the same year, the number of births with name Emmanuelle in a male is 5.*

▶ ♀**Emmeline:** From an Old French form of the Germanic name Amelina, originally a diminutive of Germanic names beginning with the element amal meaning "work." It may also be a variant form of Emilie (rival), formed by adding the diminutive suffix -ine: hence, "little rival."

**Pronunciation:** EH-mə-liyn

*For 2017, the number of births with name Emmeline is 368, which represents 0.020 percent of total female births in 2017.*

▶ ♂**Emil, ♀Emilia or Emilio**: From the Roman family name Aemilius, which was derived from Latin aemulus meaning "rival."

**Pronunciation:** eh-MEEL, AY-meel.

*For 2017, the number of births with name Emil is 142, which represents 0.007 percent of total male births in 2017.*

▶ ♂**Erdem:** Means "virtue" in Turkish.

**Pronunciation:** Eh-R-DEM

*For 2017, the number of births in the U.S. with name Erdem is less than 5.*

# LETTER F:

▶♂**Fabian:** From the Roman cognomen Fabianus, which was derived from Fabius. Saint Fabian was the 3rd-century pope.

**Pronunciation:** FAY-bee-ən

**Related to:** Fabia, Fabiano, Fabiola.

*For 2017, the number of births with name Fabian is 819, which represents 0.042 percent of total male births in 2017.*

▶♂**Fabrice:** French form of the Roman family name Fabricius, which was derived from Latin "faber" craftsman.

**Pronounced:** FAB-REES.

*For 2017, the number of births with name Fabrice is 8, which represents 0.0004 percent of total male births in 2017.*

▶♀**Faustine:** French feminine form of Faustinus (see Faustino)

**Pronunciation:** fow-STEE-ne

*For 2017, the number of female births in the U.S. with name Faustine is less than 5.*

▶♂**Faustino:** Spanish, Italian and Portuguese form of the Roman cognomen Faustinus, which was itself derived from the Roman name Faustus. Faustinus was the name of several early saints.

**Pronunciation:** FOWS-tee-noh.

*For 2017, the number of births with name Faustino is 28, which represents 0.0015 percent of total male births in 2017.*

▶♂**Felipe:** Spanish and Brazilian Portuguese form of Philip, from the Greek Philippos which means "friend of horses."

**Pronunciation:** feh-LEE-pay

*For 2017, the number of births with name Felipe is 298, which represents 0.015 percent of total male births in 2017.*

▶♂**Ferdinand:** From Ferdinando, the old Spanish form of a Germanic name composed of the elements farði "journey" and nanð "daring, brave."

**Pronunciation:** FER-di-nand

**Related to:** Fernanda, Fernando, Hernan, Ferdinardo.

*For 2017, the number of births with name Ferdinand is 17, which represents 0.0009 percent of total male births in 2017.*

▶♀♂**Finlay or Finley:** Anglicized form of Fionnlagh, and Fionnla, compound names composed of the Gaelic elements Fionn (white, fair) and laogh (warrior, calf): hence, "fair-haired warrior."

**Pronunciation:** FIN-lee

*For 2017, the number of births with name Finlay is 55, which represents 0.003 percent of total male births in 2017 and 19 female births with the same name for this year.*

▶♀**Fiona:** Feminine form of Fionn, (older Irish Finn) meaning "fair" or "white." Scottish poet James Macpherson first used this name in his poem Fingal.

**Pronounced:** fee-O-nə

*For 2017, the number of births with name Fiona is 1672, which represents 0.089 percent of total female births in 2017.*

▶♂**Flynn:** From an Irish surname, an Anglicized form of Ó Floinn meaning "descendant of FLANN." The name is derived from Flann (red): hence, "red-haired one."

**Pronunciation:** FLIN

*For 2017, the number of births with name Flynn is 309, which represents 0.0011 percent of total male births in 2017 and 19 female births with the same name for this year.*

▶♂**Foster:** From a variant of the occupational surname "Forester," belonging to a keeper of a forest or scissor maker, derived from Old French forcetier or a woodworker, derived from Old French fustrier.

**Pronunciation:** FAHS-ter

*For 2017, the number of births with name Foster is 222, which represents 0.011 percent of total male births in 2017.*

▶♀♂**Frankie:** Diminutive of Frances, the Feminine form of Francis. The distinction between Francis as a masculine name and Frances as a feminine name did not arise until the 17th century.

**Alternate versions:** Fan, Fannie, Fanny, Fran, France, Francie, Frank, Frankie, Franky, Frannie, Franny, Sis.

*For 2017, the number of births with name Frankie is 236, which represents 0.012 percent of total male births in 2017.*

*For 2017, the number of births with name Frankie is 320, which represents 0.017 percent of total female births in 2017.*

▶♀**Freja:** Danish and Swedish form of FREYA. From Old Norse Freyja meaning "lady." This was the name of the goddess of love, beauty, war, and death in Norse mythology.

**Pronounced:** FRAY-ah, FRIE-ah

**Related to:** Freyja, Frey, Frej.

*For 2017, the number of births with name Freja is 40, which represents 0.023 percent of total female births in 2017*

*"Each generation wants new symbols, new people, new names. They want to divorce themselves from their predecessors."*

JIM MORRISON

# CHAPTER 2. UNIQUE BABY NAMES G TO L

## LETTER G:

▶♂**Gabe:** Short form of Gabriel, from the Hebrew name Gavri'el meaning "strong man of God." Gabriel was one of the seven archangels in Hebrew tradition. According to Islamic tradition, he was the angel who dictated the Qur'an to Muhammad.

**Pronunciation:** GAYB

*For 2017, the number of births with name Gabe is 57, which represents 0.0031 percent of total male births in 2017*

▶♂**Gavino or Gabino:** From the Late Latin name Gabinus which meant "of Gabium." Gabium was a city of ancient Italy. Saint Gavino was martyred in Sardinia in the 2nd century.

**Pronunciation:** gah-VEE-noh

*For 2017, the number of births with name Gavino is 22, which represents 0.0012 percent of total male births in 2017.*

▶♀**Gaia:** Means "earth" in Greek. In Greek mythology, Gaia was the mother goddess who presided over the earth.

**Pronunciation:** GIY-ə

*For 2017, the number of births with name Gaia is 90, which represents 0.053 percent of total female births in 2017.*

▶♂**Gaius:** Roman praenomen, or given name, of uncertain meaning. It is possibly derived from Latin gaudere "to rejoice", though it may be of unknown Etruscan origin. This was a very common Roman praenomen, the most famous bearers being Gaius Julius Caesar.

**Pronounced:** GA-ee-oos

*For 2017, the number of births with name Gaius is 28, which represents 0.0015 percent of total male births in 2017.*

▶♀♂**Galen:** Modern form of the Greek name Γαληνος (Galenos), which meant "calm" from Greek γαληνη (galene). Derived from the name Claudius Galenus (c. 130-200), a Greek physician and writer on medicine and philosophy.

**Pronunciation:** GAY-lin

For 2017, the number of births with name Galen is 55, which represents 0.003 percent of total male births in 2017 and five female births with the same name for this year.

▶♂**Gaspar:** Latin, Spanish and Portuguese form of Jasper, "treasurer" in Persian.

**Pronounced:** ga-SPAR

**Related to:** Jasper, Casper.

*For 2017, the number of births with name Gaspar is 32, which represents 0.0017 percent of total male births in 2017.*

▶♀**Gemma:** Medieval Italian nickname meaning "gem, precious stone." It was borne by the wife of the 13th-century Italian poet Dante Alighieri.

**Pronounced:** JEM-ma.

*For 2017, the number of births with name Gemma is 1241, which represents 0.066 percent of total female births in 2017.*

▶♀**Georgina:** Feminine form of George, From the Greek name Γεωργιος (Georgios) which was derived from the Greek word γεωργος (georgos) meaning "farmer, earthworker," itself derived from the elements γη (ge) "earth" and εργον (ergon) "work."

**Pronunciation:** johr-GEE-nə

**Related to:** Georgia, Georgiana, Georgine, George, Jorge, Gigi.

*For 2017, the number of births with name Georgina is 146, which represents 0.0085 percent of total female births in 2017.*

▶ ♀**Geraldine:** Feminine form of Gerald, derived from the Germanic Gerward, a compound name composed from the elements ger (a spear) and wald (rule): hence, "spear ruler, to rule with a spear."

**Pronunciation:** jehr-əl-DEEN

*For 2017, the number of births with name Geraldine is 132, which represents 0.0077 percent of total female births in 2017.*

▶ ♂**Geronimo:** Italian form of Jerome, from the Greek name Ἱερωνυμος (Hieronymos) meaning "sacred name."

**Pronunciation:** jə-RAH-nee-moh

*For 2017, the number of births with name Geronimo is 39, which represents 0.0021 percent of total male births in 2017.*

▶ ♀**Gia:** Diminutive of Gianna or Giovanna, the feminine form of Giovanni, the Italian form of Iohannes or John ("YAHWEH is gracious").

**Related to:** Gianna, Giovanna, Giovanni and John.

*For 2017, the number of births with name Gia is 776, which represents 0.041 percent of total female births in 2017.*

▶♀**Gillian:** Medieval English feminine form of Julian, from the Roman name Iulianus, which was derived from Julius, Greek ιουλος (ioulos) "downy-bearded." Gillian was bestowed upon males and females alike. Now, however, it is an almost exclusively female name.

**Pronunciation:** JI-lee-ən, GI-lee-ən

*For 2017, the number of births with name Gillian is 81, which represents 0.0047 percent of total female births in 2017.*

▶♀**Giovanna:** See Gia.

**Pronunciation:** joh-VAHN-ə

*For 2017, the number of births with name Giovanna is 329, which represents 0.018 percent of total female births in 2017.*

▶♀**Giselle:** Derived from the Germanic word gisil meaning "hostage" or "pledge". This name may have originally been a descriptive nickname for a child given as a pledge to a foreign court.

**Pronunciation:** ji-ZEHL

*For 2017, the number of births with name Giselle is 1170, which represents 0.062 percent of total female births in 2017.*

▶♀**Giulia:** Italian feminine form of Julius, see Gillian.

**Pronounced:** JOO-lya

*For 2017, the number of births with name Giulia is 139, which represents 0.081 percent of total female births in 2017.*

▶♀♂**Gray:** From an English surname meaning "grey", originally given to a person who had grey hair or clothing.

**Pronunciation:** GRAY

*For 2017, the number of births with name Gray is 144, which represents 0.078 percent of total male births in 2017.*

*For 2017, the number of births with name Gray is 35, which represents 0.002 percent of total female births in 2017.*

▶♀♂**Greer:** From a Scottish surname which was derived from the given name Gregor.

**Pronunciation:** GREER

*For 2017, the number of births with name Greer is 89, which represents 0.0052 percent of total female births in 2017.*

*For 2017, the number of births with name Greer is 16, which represents 0.0008 percent of total male births in 2017.*

▶ ♀**Guinevere:** From the Norman French form of the Welsh name Gwenhwyfar, composed of the elements gwen meaning "fair, white" and hwyfar meaning "smooth." In Arthurian legend, she was the beautiful wife of King Arthur who engaged in an adulterous affair with Sir Lancelot.

**Pronunciation:** GWI-neh-veer

**Related to:** Geneva, Ginevra, Jennifer, Genevra

*For 2017, the number of births with name Guinevere is 190, which represents 0.011 percent of total female births in 2017.*

▶ ♀**Gwen:** From Welsh gwen, the feminine form of gwyn meaning "white, fair, blessed." It can also be a short form of Gwendolen, Gwenllian, and other names beginning with Gwen.

**Pronunciation:** GWEHN

**Related to:** Gwendolyn

*For 2017, the number of births with name Gwen is 315, which represents 0.017 percent of total female births in 2017.*

# LETTER H:

▶♂**Haden:** From Hayden, transferred use of the English surname derived from several place-names. It is from the Old English elements hēg (hay) and denu (valley); hēg (hay) and dun (hill); and hege (hedge) and dun (hill). Alternatively, the name is from the Irish Gaelic ÓhÉideáin and ÓhÉidín (descendant of Eideán or Éidín). The names are derived from éideadh (clothing).

**Pronunciation:** HA-dən.

*For 2017, the number of births with name Haden is 37, which represents 0.002 percent of total male births in 2017.*

▶♂**Hamish:** Anglicized form of a Sheumais, the vocative case of Seumas, the Scottish form of James and Jacob (supplanter).

**Pronunciation:** HAY-mish.

*For 2017, the number of births with name Hamish is 25, which represents 0.0014 percent of total male births in 2017.*

▶♂**Hamlet:** Anglicized form of the Danish name Amleth. Shakespeare used this name for the Prince of Denmark in his play 'Hamlet' (1600), which he based upon earlier Danish tales.

**Pronunciation:** HAM-leht

*For 2017, the number of births with name Hamlet is 7, which represents 0.00038 percent of total male births in 2017.*

▶♂**Han:** Variant of John (Short form of Johannes or Hans). A bearer of this name is Han Solo a hero from the 'Star Wars' movies.

**Pronounced:** HAHN.

*For 2017, the number of births with name Greer is 17, which represents 0.0009 percent of total male births in 2017.*

▶♂**Hansel:** English form of Hänsel, the German diminutive of Hans, the short form of JOHANNES (Ioannes), see Gia.

**Pronounced:** HAN-səl

*For 2017, the number of births with name Hansel is 78, which represents 0.0043 percent of total male births in 2017.*

▶♂**Harlan:** From a surname which was from a place name meaning "hare land" in Old English.

**Pronunciation:** HAR-lən

*For 2017, the number of births with name Harlan is 296, which represents 0.015 percent of total male births in 2017.*

*For 2017, the number of births with name Harlan is 34, which represents 0.002 percent of total female births in 2017.*

▶ ♀♂**Harlow:** From a surname which was from a place name which was derived from Old English hær "rock" or here "army" combined with hlaw "hill."

**Pronunciation:** HAR-loh

*For 2017, the number of births with name Harlow is 794, which represents 0.042 percent of total female births in 2017.*

*For 2017, the number of births with name Harlow is 38, which represents 0.0021 percent of total male births in 2017.*

▶ ♀♂**Haven:** From the English word for a safe place, derived ultimately from Old English hæfen.

**Pronunciation:** HAY-vin.

**Related to:** Heaven and Heavenly.

*For 2017, the number of births with name Haven is 1080, which represents 0.058 percent of total female births in 2017.*

*For 2017, the number of births with name Haven is 115, which represents 0.0063 percent of total male births in 2017.*

▶♂**Henson:** Transferred use of the surname Henson.

**Pronunciation:** HEN-son.

*For 2017, the number of births with name Henson is 19, which represents 0.001 percent of total male births in 2017.*

▶♀**Hera:** Uncertain meaning, possibly from Greek 'ηρως (heros) "hero, warrior," 'ωρα (hora) "period of time," or 'αιρεω (haireo) "to be chosen." In Greek mythology, Hera was the queen of the gods, the sister, and wife of Zeus. She presided over marriage and childbirth.

**Pronounced:** HE-RA

*For 2017, the number of births with name Hera is 37, which represents 0.0022 percent of total female births in 2017.*

▶♀**Hermione:** Derived from the name of the Greek messenger god Hermes. In Greek myth, Hermione was the daughter of Menelaus and Helen.

**Pronunciation:** her-MIY-ə-nee.

*For 2017, the number of births with name Hermione is 80, which represents 0.0047 percent of total female births in 2017.*

► ♀♂**Honor:** Derived from the Latin honor (esteem, integrity, dignity).

**Pronunciation:** AW-ner.

*For 2017, the number of births with name Honor is 105, which represents 0.0061 percent of total female births in 2017.*

*For 2017, the number of births with name Honor is 98, which represents 0.0053 percent of total male births in 2017.*

# LETTER I:

►♂**Iago:** Welsh and Galician form of Jacob, from the Latin Iacobus, which was from the Greek Ιακωβος (Iakobos), which was from the Hebrew name Ya'aqov. In the Old Testament, Jacob (later called Israel) is the son of Isaac and Rebecca and the father of the twelve founders of the twelve tribes of Israel. He was born holding his twin brother Esau's heel, and his name is explained as meaning "holder of the heel" or "supplanter."

**Pronounced:** ee-AH-go

*For 2017, the number of male births with name Iago is less than 5.*

►♂**Ichiro:** Variant transcription of Ichirou, From Japanese 一 (ichi) "one" and 郎 (rou) "son." This was traditionally a name given to the first son.

**Pronounced:** EE-CHEE-RO

*For 2017, the number of male births with name Iago is 6.*

►♂**Idan:** Means "era or time" in Hebrew

**Pronunciation:** EE - don

*For 2017, the number of births with name Idan is 21, which represents 0.0011 percent of total male births in 2017.*

► ♀♂**Ilan:** Means "tree" in Hebrew.

**Pronunciation:** i-LAHN

*For 2017, the number of births with name Ilan is 114, which represents 0.0062 percent of total male births in 2017, and a total of 5 female births for the same year.*

► ♀**Ilaria:** Italian feminine form of Hilarius. From the Greek word 'ιλαρος (hilaris) meaning "cheerful."

**Pronunciation:** ee-LAH-ree-ə

*For 2017, the number of births with name Ilaria is 34, which represents 0.002 percent of total female births in 2017.*

► ♀**Iliana:** Variant of Ileana, possibly a Romanian variant of Helen. In Romanian folklore, this is the name of a princess kidnapped by monsters and rescued by a heroic knight.

**Related to**: Ileana and Helen.

*For 2017, the number of births with name Iliana is 292, which represents 0.016 percent of total female births in 2017.*

► ♀**Ilsa or Ilse:** German and Dutch diminutive of Elisabeth/ Elizabeth, from Ελισαβετ (Elisabet), the Greek form of the Hebrew name Elisheba meaning "my God is an oath" or perhaps "my God is abundance."

**Pronunciation:** IL-sə

*For 2017, the number of births with name Ilsa is 18, which represents 0.0011 percent of total female births in 2017.*

▶♀♂**Iman:** Means "faith," derived from Arabic Amuna "to be faithful."

**Pronunciation:** EE-MON

*For 2017, the number of births with name Iman is 105, which represents 0.0061 percent of total female births in 2017.*

*For 2017, the number of births with name Iman is 40, which represents 0.0022 percent of total male births in 2017.*

▶♂**Imanol:** Basque form of Emmanuel, from the Hebrew name 'Immanu'el meaning "God, is with us."

**Pronunciation:** ee-maa-nohl

*For 2017, the number of births with name Imanol is 7, which represents 0.0003 percent of total male births in 2017.*

▶♀**Imogen:** The name of a princess in the play Cymbeline by Shakespeare. He based her on a legendary character named Innogen, a Celtic name supposedly derived from the Gaelic inghean (girl, maiden), but the name was printed incorrectly and never corrected.

**Pronunciation:** IM-oh-jehn

*For 2017, the number of births with name Imogen is 169, which represents 0.0099 percent of total female births in 2017.*

▶ ♀**Inaya:** is an indirect Quranic name for girls that means "help," "care," "protection." It is derived from the Ain-W-N root which is used in many places in the Quran,

**Pronounced:** in-NAY-a

**Similar to:** Inayya, Inaya, Iynaayah, Naya.

*For 2017, the number of births with name Inaya is 131, which represents 0.0077 percent of total female births in 2017.*

▶ ♀**Indira:** Means "beauty" in Sanskrit. This is another name of Lakshmi, the wife of the Hindu god Vishnu.

**Pronounced:** ihn-DEE-raa

*For 2017, the number of births with name Imdira is 41, which represents 0.0024 percent of total female births in 2017.*

▶ ♀**Isadora:** Variant of Isidora, female of Isidore, from the Greek name Ισιδωρος (Isidoros) which meant "gift of Isis," derived from the name of the Egyptian goddess Isis combined with Greek δωρον (doron) "gift".

**Related to:** Isidore, Isador, Issy, Izzy. Isidro.

**Pronounced:** IZA-dawra

*For 2017, the number of births with name Isadora is 14, which represents 0.0007 percent of total female births in 2017.*

▶ ♀**Ishana:** Female form of Indian name Ishan, Derived from Sanskrit ईश् (īś) meaning "master, lord".

**Related to:** Ishan, Ishaan, Ishani

**Prononced:** E-sh-aa-na

*For 2017, the number of births with name Ishana is 21, which represents 0.0012 percent of total female births in 2017.*

▶ ♂**Ishmael:** From the Hebrew name Yishma'el meaning "God will hear." In the Old Testament, this is the name of a son of Abraham. He is the traditional ancestor of the Arabs.

**Pronunciation:** ISH-miy-ehl

*For 2017, the number of births with name Ishmael is 155, which represents 0.0084 percent of total male births in 2017.*

► ♀**Ivette:** Spanish form of Yvette, the feminine form of Yves, the Medieval French form of Ivo meaning "yew."

**Pronunciation:** EE-veht

*For 2017, the number of births with name Ivette is 67, which represents 0.0039 percent of total female births in 2017.*

# LETTER J:

▶♂**Jacques:** French form of Jacob ("supplanter") or James.

**Pronunciation:** ZHAHK

**Related to:** Jacob, James, Jacobus, Jimmie, Jimmy, Jacqueline, Jacquette.

*For 2017, the number of births with name Jacques is 66, which represents 0.0036 percent of total male births in 2017.*

▶♂**Jaeger or Jagger:** Anglicized spelling of the German surname Jäger, itself from the Middle High German jeger(e) meaning "hunter."

**Pronunciation:** YAE-ger

*For 2017, the number of births with name Jaeger is 28, which represents 0.0015 percent of total male births in 2017.*

▶♂**Jair:** Means "he shines" in Hebrew. In the Old Testament, this is the name of both a son of Manasseh and one of the judges of the Israelites.

**Pronunciation:** JAYR, JAY-er

*For 2017, the number of births with name Jair is 178, which represents 0.0097 percent of total male births in 2017.*

►♂**Jared:** From the Hebrew name Yared or Yered meaning "descent." This is the name of a close descendent of Adam in the Old Testament.

**Pronunciation:** JEH-rid, JA-rid

*For 2017, the number of births with name Jared is 839, which represents 0.043 percent of total male births in 2017.*

►♂**Jarrett:** From a surname which was a variant of Garrett

**Pronunciation:** JA-rit

For 2017, the number of births with name Jarrett is 140, which represents 0.0076 percent of total male births in 2017.

►♂**Jarvis:** From a surname which was derived from the given name Gervais or Gervasius, derived from Germanic word ger "spear."

**Pronounced:** JAHR-vis

*For 2017, the number of births with name Jarvis is 119, which represents 0.0065 percent of total male births in 2017.*

►♂**Javen:** probably related to Javan which means "Greece" in Hebrew.

**Pronounced:** JA-VIN

*For 2017, the number of births with name Javen is 70, which represents 0.0038 percent of total male births in 2017.*

## ▶♀Jemima or Jemina: Means "dove" in Hebrew. This was the oldest of the three daughters of Job in the Old Testament.

**Pronounced:** jə-MIE-mə

For 2017, the number of births with name Jemima is 38, which represents 0.0022 percent of total female births in 2017.

## ▶♀Jemma: Variant of Gemma

**Pronunciation:** JEH-mə

*For 2017, the number of births with name Jemma is 491, which represents 0.026 percent of total female births in 2017.*

## ▶♀Jezebel: From the Hebrew 'Izevel which meant "not exalted." In the Old Testament, this is the name of the evil wife of Ahab, king of Israel.

**Pronunciation:** JEH-zə-behl

*For 2017, the number of births with name Jezebel is 27, which represents 0.0016 percent of total female births in 2017.*

## ▶♀Jillian: Variant of Gillian

**Pronunciation:** JI-lee-in

*For 2017, the number of births with name Jillian is 523, which represents 0.028 percent of total female births in 2017.*

▶♀**Jimena:** Variant of Ximena, the feminine of Ximeno, from medieval Spanish or Basque name of uncertain meaning, possibly a form of Simon, though it may derive from Basque seme meaning "son".

**Pronunciation:** hee-MEH-nah

*For 2017, the number of births with name Jimena is 772, which represents 0.041 percent of total female births in 2017.*

▶♀**Jolie:** Means "pretty" in French

**Pronunciation:** JOH-lee, joh-LEE

*For 2017, the number of births with name Jolie is 437, which represents 0.023 percent of total female births in 2017.*

▶♀**Jules:** Diminutive of Julia or Julian, the Feminine form of Julius "downy-bearded" or related to Jupiter.

**Pronounced:** ZHUYL or JOOLZ

*For 2017, the number of births with name Jules is 112, which represents 0.0065 percent of total female births in 2017.*

▶♀**Julianne:** Feminine form of Iulianus (see Jules)

*For 2017, the number of births with name Julianne is 205, which represents 0.012 percent of total female births in 2017.*

▶♀**Juliet:** Anglicized form of Juliette or Giulietta. Shakespeare first used this spelling for the lover of Romeo in his play Romeo and Juliet.

**Pronunciation:** joo-lee-EHT.

**Related to:** Giulia, Giulietta, Julie, Juliette.

*For 2017, the number of births with name Juliet is 1378, which represents 0.073 percent of total female births in 2017.*

▶♀**Juniper:** From the English word for the type of tree, derived ultimately from Latin iuniperus

Pronunciation: JOO-ni-per

*For 2017, the number of births with name Juniper is 1033, which represents 0.055 percent of total female births in 2017.*

# LETTER K:

▶♂**Kade:** Variant of Cade, derived from a surname which was originally derived from a nickname meaning "round, cask or barrel" in Old English.

**Related to:** Cade, Caden, Kaden, Kaiden.

**Pronunciation:** KAYD

*For 2017, the number of births with name Kade is 748, which represents 0.038 percent of total male births in 2017.*

▶♂**Kahlil:** Variant of Khalil (Friend in Arabic)

**Related to:** Khaleel or Khalil

*For 2017, the number of births with name Kahlil is 83, which represents 0.0045 percent of total male births in 2017.*

▶♀**Kaia:** A variant of Kaja, a Scandinavian diminutive of Katarina. It could also be derived from Old Norse kaða meaning "hen" or Derived from the Hawaiian kai (the sea).

**Pronunciation:** KIY-ə

*For 2017, the number of births with name Kaia is 978, which represents 0.052 percent of total female births in 2017.*

►♂**Kale:** Hawaiian form of Charles, From the Germanic name Karl, which was derived from a Germanic word which meant "man." However, an alternative theory states that it is derived from the common Germanic element hari meaning "army, warrior."

**Related to:** Charles.

**Pronunciation:** KAYL

For 2017, the number of births with name Kale is 61, which represents 0.0063 percent of total male births in 2017.

►♀**Kali:** Means "the black one" in Sanskrit. The Hindu goddess Kali is the fierce destructive form of the wife of Shiva.

**Pronunciation:** KAH-lee

*For 2017, the number of births with name Kali is 1083, which represents 0.058 percent of total female births in 2017.*

►♀**Kalliope:** Means "beautiful voice" from Greek καλλος (kallos) "beauty" and οψ (ops) "voice." In Greek mythology, she was a goddess of epic poetry and eloquence, one of the nine Muses.

**Pronunciation:** kə-LIY-oh-pee

*For 2017, the number of births with name Kalliope is 76, which represents 0.0044 percent of total female births in 2017.*

▶ ♀♂**Kamari:** Likely a variant of Kamaria, Swahili for Qamar, means "moon" in Arabic.

**Pronounced:** Kee-MA-ree

*For 2017, the number of births with name Kamari is 422, which represents 0.021 percent of total male births in 2017.*

*For 2017, the number of births with name Kamari is 252, which represents 0.015 percent of total female births in 2017.*

▶ ♀**Karmen:** Slovene and Croatian form of Carmen, Medieval Spanish form of Carmel influenced by the Latin word carmen "song" or of Carmel (vineyard, orchard)

**Pronunciation:** KAHR-min

*For 2017, the number of births with name karmen is 191, which represents 0.0011 percent of total female births in 2017.*

▶ ♀**Kamilla:** Hungarian and Scandinavian form of the Latin name Camilla (virgin of unblemished character).

**Similar to:** Camilla, Camille, Kamille.

**Pronunciation:** kah-MIL-ə

*For 2017, the number of births with name Kamilla is 169, which represents 0.0099 percent of total female births in 2017.*

▶♂**Kaspar:** form of Jasper, see Caspar.

**Pronounced:** KAS-par

*For 2017, the number of male births with name Kaspar is less than 5.*

▶♀**Katarina:** Cognate of Katherine, from the Greek name Αικατερινη (Aikaterine). The etymology is debated: it could derive from the earlier Greek name Ἑκατερινη (Hekaterine), which came from ἑκατερο\[FinalSigma] (hekateros) "each of the two"; it could derive from the name of the goddess Hecate; it could be related to Greek αικια (aikia) "torture"; or it could be from a Coptic name meaning "my consecration of your name".

**Pronunciation:** kah-teh-REE-nə

*For 2017, the number of births with name Katarina is 141, which represents 0.0082 percent of total female births in 2017.*

▶♀**Kayley:** Variant of Kaylee, a combination of Kay and the popular name suffix lee.

**Pronunciation:** KAY-lee

*For 2017, the number of births with name Kayley is 100, which represents 0.0058 percent of total female births in 2017.*

## ►♂Keagan or Keegan: Transferred use of the Anglicized surname, which is from MacAodhagáin (son of Aodhagán). The name Aodhagán is a double diminutive form of Aodh (fire); hence, "little fire."

**Pronunciation:** KEE-gən

*For 2017, the number of births with name Keagan is 245, which represents 0.012 percent of total male births in 2017.*

## ►♂Keane: Variant of Kean, the Anglicized form of Cian, which means "ancient" in Gaelic. This was the name of the mythical ancestor of the Cianachta in Irish legend.

**Related to:** Kean and Cian.

**Pronunciation:** KEEN

*For 2017, the number of births with name Keane is 31, which represents 0.0017 percent of total male births in 2017.*

## ►♂Keanu: Possibly means "cool breeze" in Hawaiian

**Pronunciation:** keh-AH-noo

*For 2017, the number of births with name Keanu is 238, which represents 0.012 percent of total male births in 2017.*

▶♀**Keeley:** Variant of Keely, from an Irish surname, an Anglicized form of Ó Caolaidhe meaning "descendent of Caoladhe". The given name Caoladhe is derived from the Gaelic word caol "slender".

**Pronunciation:** KEE-lee

*For 2017, the number of births with name Keeley is 84, which represents 0.0049 percent of total female births in 2017.*

▶♀**Keila:** Possibly a variant of Kayla, Yiddish form of Kelila, that means "crown of laurel" in Hebrew.

**Related to:** Kayla and Kyla.

**Pronounced:** KAY-LA or KEE-la

*For 2017, the number of births with name Keyla is 345, which represents 0.018 percent of total female births in 2017.*

▶♂**Kenji:** From Japanese 研 (ken) "study" and 二 (ji) "two" (as well as other combinations of kanji characters). Also, may be a short form or Kenjiro or Kenjirou.

**Pronounced:** KEN-"gee"

*For 2017, the number of births with name Kenji is 136, which represents 0.034 percent of total male births in 2017.*

► ♂**Khalid:** Means "eternal", derived from Arabic khalada "to last forever"

**Pronunciation:** kah-LEED

*For 2017, the number of births with name Khalid is 253, which represents 0.013 percent of total male births in 2017.*

► ♂**Kilian:** Irish variant and German form of Cillian, probably from Gaelic ceall "church" combined with a diminutive suffix. This was the name of a 7th-century Irish saint who evangelized Franconia.

**Pronunciation:** KIL-ee-ən

*For 2017, the number of births with name Kilian is 162, which represents 0.0088 percent of total male births in 2017.*

► ♀**Kyla:** Feminine form of Kyle, from a Scottish surname which was derived from Gaelic caol meaning "narrows, channel, strait".

**Pronunciation:** KIY-lə

*For 2017, the number of births with name Kyla is 802, which represents 0.043 percent of total female births in 2017.*

# LETTER L:

▶♀**Lainey**: Variant of Laney, diminutive of Elaine, from an Old French variant of Helen, English form of the Greek 'Ελενη (Helene), probably from Greek 'ελενη (helene) "torch" or "corposant" or possibly related to σεληνη (selene) "moon".

**Pronunciation:** LAY-nee

*For 2017, the number of births with name Lainey is 610, which represents 0.033 percent of total female births in 2017.*

▶♂**Landen:** Variant of Landon, from a surname which was derived from an Old English place name meaning "long hill".

**Pronunciation:** LAN-dən

*For 2017, the number of births with name Landen is 746, which represents 0.038 percent of total male births in 2017.*

▶♀**Lani:** Means "sky, heaven" in Hawaiian.

**Pronunciation:** LAH-nee

*For 2017, the number of births with name Lani is 78, which represents 0.046 percent of total female births in 2017.*

▶♀**Larissa or Larisa:** Possibly derived from the name of the ancient city of Larisa in Thessaly, which meant "citadel". In Greek mythology, the nymph Larisa was a daughter of Pelasgus. This name was later borne by a 4th-century Greek martyr who is venerated as a saint in the Eastern Church.

**Pronunciation:** lah-RIS-ə

*For 2017, the number of births with name Larissa is 205, which represents 0.012 percent of total female births in 2017.*

▶♀**Lavinia:** Meaning unknown, probably of Etruscan origin. In Roman legend Lavinia was the daughter of King Latinus, the wife of Aeneas, and the ancestor of the Roman people.

**Pronunciation:** lah-VIN-ee-ə

*For 2017, the number of births with name Lavinia is 67, which represents 0.0039 percent of total female births in 2017.*

▶♂**Lazarus:** Latinized form of Λαζαρος (Lazaros), a Greek form of Eleazar. Lazarus was a man who was restored to life by Jesus.

**Pronunciation:** LA-zə-ruhs.

*For 2017, the number of births with name Lazarus is 151, which represents 0.0082 percent of total male births in 2017.*

▶♂**Leandro:** Spanish, Portuguese and Italian form of Leander, from the Greek Λεανδρος (Leandros) which means "lion of a man" from Greek λεων (leon) "lion" and ανδρος (andros) "of a man". In Greek legend Leander was the lover of Hero. Every night he swam across the Hellespont to meet her, but on one occasion he was drowned when a storm arose. When Hero saw his dead body, she threw herself into the waters and perished.

**Pronunciation:** leh-AHN-droh

*For 2017, the number of births with name Leandro is 333, which represents 0.017 percent of total male births in 2017.*

▶♀**Leilani:** Means "heavenly flowers" in Hawaiian, Lani (sky, heaven, heavenly, spiritual; majesty) and lei (a wreath of flowers and leaves, garland).

**Pronunciation:** lay-LAH-nee

*For 2017, the number of births with name Leilani is 2264, which represents 0.121 percent of total female births in 2017.*

▶♂**Leopold:** Derived from the Germanic elements leud "people" and bald "bold". The spelling was altered due to association with Latin leo"lion".

**Pronunciation:** LEE-ə-pohld.

*For 2017, the number of births with name Leopold is 105, which represents 0.0057 percent of total male births in 2017.*

▶♂**Lex:** Short form of Alexander, latinized form of the Greek name Αλεξανδρος (Alexandros), which meant "defending men" from Greek αλεξω (alexo)"to defend, help" and ανδρος (andros) genitive form of "man".

**Pronunciation:** LEHKS

*For 2017, the number of births with name Lex is 90, which represents 0.0049 percent of total male births in 2017*

▶♀**Libby:** Originally a medieval diminutive of Ibb, itself a diminutive of Isabel. It is also used as a diminutive of Elizabeth ("my God is an oath" or perhaps "my God is abundance").

**Pronunciation:** LI-bee

*For 2017, the number of births with name Libby is 237, which represents 0.014 percent of total female births in 2017.*

▶♀**Lissandra:** Derived from the Greek Alexandros, a male compound name composed of the elements alexein (to defend, to help) and andros (man).

**Pronounced:** lih-SAHN-drah

*For 2017, the number of births with name Lissandra is 12, which represents 0.0007 percent of total female births in 2017.*

▶♀**Liv:** Derived from the Old Norse name Hlíf meaning "protection". Its use has been influenced by the modern Scandinavian word liv meaning "life". Short form of Olivia

**Pronunciation:** LIV

*For 2017, the number of births with name Liv is 432, which represents 0.023 percent of total female births in 2017.*

▶♀**Lorelei:** From a Germanic name meaning "luring rock". Legends say that a maiden named the Lorelei lives on the rock and lures fishermen to their death with her song.

**Pronunciation:** LOH-rə-liy

*For 2017, the number of births with name Lorelei is 680, which represents 0.036 percent of total female births in 2017.*

▶♀**Lourdes:** From the name of a French town, a popular center of Christian pilgrimage. Transferred use of a Basque place-name meaning "craggy slope."

**Pronunciation:** LOOR-dəs, LUWRDZ.

*For 2017, the number of births with name Lourdes is 91, which represents 0.0053 percent of total female births in 2017.*

►♂**Lucian:** Romanian and English form of Lucianus or Lucius a roman given name which was derived from Latin lux "light."

**Pronunciation:** LOO-shən

*For 2017, the number of births with name Lucian is 462, which represents 0.024 percent of total male births in 2017.*

►♀**Lyra:** The name of the constellation in the northern sky containing the star Vega. It is said to be shaped after the lyre of Orpheus.

**Pronunciation:** LIY-rə

*For 2017, the number of births with name Lyra is 390, which represents 0.021 percent of total female births in 2017.*

*"People's fates are simplified by their names."*


ELIAS CANETTI,

GERMAN-LANGUAGE AUTHOR, BORN IN RUSE, BULGARIA

# CHAPTER 3. **UNIQUE BABY NAMES M TO R**

## LETTER M:

▶♂**Mace:** Male nickname for Mason, a name of English origin meaning "one who works with stone."

**Pronunciation:** Mays

*The number of births with name Mace is 46, which represents 0.0005 percent of total male births in 2017.*

▶♂*Maurizio:* Male name derived from the Roman name Mauritius, a derivative of MAURUS, which means "dark-skinned". Related to Maurice

**Pronunciation:** *mow-REE-tsyo*

*The number of births with name Maurizio is 46, which represents 0.0005 percent of total male births in 2017.*

▶♀**Magdalene:** From a title which meant "of Magdala". Mary Magdalene, a character in the New Testament, was named thus because she was from Magdala, a village on the Sea of Galilee whose name meant "tower" in Hebrew. She was a popular saint in the Middle Ages, and the name became common then.

Pronunciation: MAG-də-leen

*The number of births with name Magdalene is 109, which represents 0.0064 percent of total female births in 2017.*

### ▶♀Marion: Medieval French diminutive of Marie

**Pronunciation:** MER-ee-ən

*The number of births with name Marion is 141, which represents 0.0082 percent of total female births in 2017.*

### ▶♂Maximilian: From the Roman name Maximilianus, which was derived from MAXIMUS. In the 15th century, the Holy Roman emperor Frederick III gave this name to his son and eventual heir. In this case, it was a blend of the names of the Roman generals Fabius Maximus and Cornelius Scipio Aemilianus.

**Pronunciation:** mak-sə-MIL-yən

*The number of births with name Maximilian is 647, which represents 0.033 percent of total male births in 2017.*

### ▶♀Matilda: From the Germanic name Mahthildis meaning "strength in battle," from the elements maht "might, strength" and hild "battle." Saint Matilda was the wife of the 10th-century German king Henry I the Fowler. The name was common in many branches of European royalty in the Middle Ages. It was brought

to England by the Normans, being borne by the wife of William the Conqueror himself.

**Pronunciation:** mə-TIL-də

*The number of births with name Matilda is 597, which represents 0.035 percent of total female births in 2017.*

▶♂**Mika:** Male name from Japanese 美 (mi) meaning "beautiful" combined with 香 (ka) meaning "fragrance" or 加 (ka) meaning "increase."

Also, from the Finnish short form of Mikael.

**Pronunciation:** MEE-kah

*The number of births with name Mika is 200, which represents 0.012 percent of total male births in 2017.*

▶♀**Milena:** Feminine form of MILAN. It began to be used in Italy in honor of Milena Vukotić (1847-1923), mother of Helen of Montenegro, the wife of the Italian king Victor Emmanuel III. In Italy, it can also be considered a combination of MARIA and ELENA.

**Pronunciation:** mee-LE-na

*The number of births with name Mika is 325, which represents 0.019 percent of total female births in 2017.*

▶♀**Minerva:** Female name possibly derived from Latin mens meaning "intellect," but more likely of

Etruscan origin. Minerva was the Roman goddess of wisdom and war, approximately equivalent to the Greek goddess Athena. It has been used as a given name in the English-speaking world since after the Renaissance.

**Pronunciation:** mi-NER-və

*The number of births with name Minerva is 68, which represents 0.004 percent of total female births in 2017.*

▶♀**Moira:** Anglicized form of female name MÁIRE. It also coincides with Greek Μοιρα (Moira) meaning "fate, destiny," the singular of Μοιραι, the Greek name for the Fates. They were the three female personifications of destiny in Greek mythology.

**Pronunciation:** MOY-rə

*The number of births with name Moira is 132, which represents 0.0077 percent of total female births in 2017*

▶♂**Mordecai:** Means "servant of MARDUK" in Persian. In the Old Testament Mordecai is the cousin and foster father of Esther.

**Pronunciation**: MAWR-də-kie

The number of births with name Maximilian is 64, which represents 0.0035 percent of total male births in 2017.

►♀**Muriel:** Medieval English form of a Celtic name which was probably related to the female Irish name MUIRGEL. The Normans brought it to England from Brittany.

**Pronunciation:** MUR-ee-əl

*The number of births with name Minerva is 24, which represents 0.0014 percent of total female births in 2017.*

# LETTER N:

▶ ♀**Naiara:** Female name from the Basque name of the Spanish city of Nájera, which is Arabic in origin.

**Pronunciation:** Nay-ARR-uh

*The number of births with name Naiara is 23, which represents 0.0013 percent of total female births in 2017.*

▶ ♂**Narciso:** Italian, the Spanish and Portuguese form of Narcissus. Narcissus was a beautiful youth in Greek mythology who stared at his reflection for so long that he eventually died and was turned into the narcissus flower.

**Pronunciation:** nar-SEE-so

*The number of births with name Narciso is 12, which represents 0.00065 percent of total male births in 2017.*

▶ ♂**Nasib**: Male name meaning "noble" in Arabic.

**Pronunciation:** na-SEEB

The number of births with name Nasib is 5, which represents 0.00027 percent of total male births in 2017.

►♀**Natividad:** Female name from the Spanish word meaning "nativity," referring to the nativity of Jesus.

**Pronunciation:** nah-tee-vee-DAD

*The number of births with name Natividad is 6, which represents 0.00025 percent of total female births in 2017.*

►♀**Nereida:** Female name derived from Greek Νηρειδες (Nereides), meaning "nymphs, sea sprites", ultimately derived from the name of the Greek sea god Nereus, who supposedly fathered them.

**Pronunciation:** ne-REY-dha

*The number of births with name Nereida is 10, which represents 0.00058 percent of total female births in 2017.*

►♀*Nerissa:* Female name created by Shakespeare for a character in his play 'The Merchant of Venice.' He possibly took it from the name Nereida.

Pronunciation:

*The number of births with name Nerissa is 15, which represents 0.00088 percent of total female births in 2017.*

►♂**Neville:** Male name derived from an English surname which was originally derived from a place name meaning "new town" in Norman French. As a given name it is chiefly British and Australian.

**Pronunciation:** NEV-əl

*The number of births with name Neville is 13, which represents 0.00071 percent of total male births in 2017.*

▶♀**Niamh:** Female name Meaning "bright" in Irish. She was the daughter of the sea god in Irish legends. She fell in love with the poet Oisín, son of Fionn.

**Pronunciation:** niːəv or niːv

*The number of births with name Niamh is 37, which represents 0.0037 percent of total female births in 2017.*

▶♂**Nicola:** Italian form of NICHOLAS.

**Pronunciation:** nee-KAW-la

*The number of births with name Nicola is 26, which represents 0.0014 percent of total male births in 2017.*

▶♂**Nikita:** Russian form of Niketas derived from Greek νικητης (niketes) meaning "winner, victor". Saint Niketas was a 4th-century bishop of Remesiana in Serbia. He is the patron saint of Romania.

Pronunciation: ni-KEE-tə

*The number of births with name Nikita is 69, which represents 0.0038 percent of total male births in 2017.*

▶♀**Nissa:** a female name meaning "sign" in Hebrew.

**Pronunciation:** NIS-ə

*The number of births with name Nissa is 14, which represents 0.00082 percent of total female births in 2017.*

▶♂**Norbert**: Male name meaning light of the north. It is derived from the Germanic elements nord "north" and beraht "bright."

**Pronunciation:** NOHR-bert

*The number of births with name Norbert is 8, which represents 0.00044 percent of total male births in 2017.*

▶♂**Norval:** Derived from the surname Norval, which is an Anglo-Scottish variant of Norville, a Norman French surname that was brought to Great Britain during or after the Norman Conquest. The meaning of the name is basically "town of the Normans."

**Pronunciation:** NOR-vəl

*The number of births with name Nicola is less than 5 of total male births in 2017.*

▶ ♀ **Nuria**: From a Catalan title of the Virgin Mary, Nostra Senyora de Núria, meaning "Our Lady of Nuria." Nuria is a sanctuary in Spain in which there is a shrine containing a famous statue of Mary.

**Pronunciation**: NOO-ree-ə

*The number of births with name Nuria is 16, which represents 0.00093 percent of total female births in 2017.*

▶ ♀ **Nyoka:** Swahili word for "snake."

**Pronunciation:** NIE-o-kə

*The number of female births with name Nyoka is less than 5 in 2017.*

# LETTER O:

▶♂**Obadiah:** Male name that Means "serving YAHWEH" in Hebrew. In the Old Testament, this is the name of one of the twelve minor prophets, the author of the Book of Obadiah, which predicts the downfall of the nation of Edom.

**Pronunciation:** o-bə-DIE-ə

*The number of births with name Obadiah is 95, which represents 0.0052 percent of total male births in 2017.*

▶♀**Oda:** Feminine form of Odo, originally a short form of various names beginning with the Germanic element aud meaning "wealth, fortune".

**Pronunciation**: O-da

*The number of births with name Oda is less than 5 of total female births in 2017.*

▶♀**Odilia:** Derived from the Germanic element odal meaning "fatherland" or aud meaning "wealth, fortune". Saint Odilia (or Odila) was an 8th-century nun who is considered the patron saint of Alsace. She was born blind but gained sight when she was baptized.

**Pronunciation:** oh-DEEL-yə

*The number of births with name Odilia is less than 5 of total female births in 2017.*

▶♂**Olaf**: From the Old Norse name Áleifr meaning "ancestor's descendant", derived from the elements anu "ancestor" and leifr "descendant." This was the name of five kings of Norway, including Saint Olaf (Olaf II).

**Pronunciation:** O-laf

*The number of births with name Obadiah is 8 of the total male births in 2017.*

▶♀**Olympia:** Feminine form of Olympos, the name of the mountain home of the Greek gods.

**Pronunciation:** oh-LIM-pee-ə

*The number of births with name Olympia is 62 of total female births in 2017.*

▶♀**Oriana:** Possibly derived from Latin aurum "gold" or its derivatives, Spanish oro or French or.

**Pronunciaton:** o-RYA-na

*The number of births with name Oda is 106 of total female births in 2017.*

▶♂**Orson:** From an English surname, which was originally a nickname meaning, "bear cub," from a diminutive of Norman French ors "bear," ultimately from Latin ursus.

**Pronunciation:** AWR-sən

*The number of births with name Orson is 73 of total male births in 2017.*

▶♂**Oswald:** Derived from the Old English elements os "god" and weald "power, ruler". Though the name had died out by the end of the Middle Ages, it was revived in the 19th century. Diminutives: Oz, Ozzie, Ozzy

Pronunciation: AHZ-wawld

*The number of births with name Oswald is 38 of total male births in 2017.*

# LETTER P:

▶♂**Padraig:** Gaelic form of Patrick.

**Pronunciation:** PAW-drig

*The number of births with name Padraig is 15 of total male births in 2017.*

▶♂**Pan:** Possibly from an Indo-European root meaning "shepherd, protector." In Greek mythology, Pan was a half-man, half-goat god associated with shepherds, flocks, and pastures.

Pronunciation: PAN

*The number of births with name Philemon is less than 5 of total male births in 2017.*

▶♀**Pandora:** Means "all gifts", derived from a combination of Greek παν (pan) "all" and δωρον (doron) "gift." In Greek mythology, Pandora was the first mortal woman. Zeus gave her a jar containing all of the troubles and ills that humanity now knows and told her not to open it. Unfortunately, her curiosity got the best of her, and she opened it, unleashing the evil spirits into the world.

**Pronunciation:** pan-DAWR-ə

*The number of births with name Pandora is 53 of total female births in 2017.*

▶♀**Pascal:** From the Late Latin name Paschalis, which meant "relating to Easter" from Latin Pascha "Easter," which was in turn from Hebrew פֶּסַח (pesach) meaning "Passover". Passover is the ancient Hebrew holiday celebrating the liberation from Egypt. Because it coincided closely with the later Christian holiday of Easter, the same Latin word was used for both.

**Pronunciation:** pas-KAL

*The number of births with name Pascal is less than 5 of total female births in 2017.*

▶♀*Paz:* Means "peace" in Spanish and "gold" in Hebrew.

Pronunciation:

*The number of births with name Paz is 6 of total female births in 2017.*

▶♀**Phaedra:** From the Greek meaning "bright". Phaedra was the daughter of Minos and the wife of Theseus in Greek mythology.

**Pronunciation:** FAY-drə

*The number of births with name Phaedra is 27 of total female births in 2017.*

▶♂**Philemon:** Means "affectionate" in Greek, a derivative of philema "kiss".

Pronunciation: fie-LEE-mən

*The number of births with name Philemon is 24 of total male births in 2017.*

▶ ♀**Pia:** Feminine form of Pius. Late Latin name meaning "pious, dutiful."

**Pronunciation:** PEE-a

*The number of births with name Pia is less than 5 of total female births in 2017.*

▶ ♀**Pilar:** Means "pillar" in Spanish. It is taken from the title of the Virgin Mary, María del Pilar, meaning "Mary of the Pillar." According to legend, when Saint James the Greater was in Saragossa in Spain, the Virgin Mary appeared on a pillar.

**Pronunciation:** pee-LAR

*The number of births with name Pilar is 56 of total female births in 2017.*

▶ ♀**Portia:** Variant of Porcia, the feminine form of the Roman family name Porcious, used by William Shakespeare for the heroine of his play 'The Merchant of Venice' (1596). In the play, Portia is a woman who disguises herself as a man to defend Antonio in court.

**Pronunciation:** PAWR-shə

*The number of births with name Portia is 26 of total female births in 2017.*

▶ ♀**Phyllis:** Means "foliage" in Greek. In Greek mythology, this was the name of a woman who killed herself out of love for Demophon and was subsequently transformed into an almond tree. It began to be used as a given name in England in the 16th century.

**Pronunciation:** FI-lis

*The number of births with name Phyllis is 103 of total female births in 2017.*

# LETTER Q:

▶♂**Qadim:** Male name of Arabic origin meaning "ancient."

Pronunciation: kah-DEEM

*The number of births with name Qadim is 13 of total male births in 2017.*

▶♀**Qiana:** From 'star' in Farsi.

**Pronunciation:** kee-AH-nə

*The number of births with name Qiana is 8 of total female births in 2017.*

▶♂*Quaid:* Derived from Gaelic Mac Uaid meaning "son of Uaid,"

**Pronunciation:** *KWAYD*

*The number of births with name Quaid is 22 of total male births in 2017.*

▶♂**Quinlan:** From Irish Ó Caoindealbháin, which means "descendant of Caoindealbhán", a given name meaning "comely form."

**Pronunciation:** KWIN-lən

*The number of births with name Quinlan is 51 of total male births in 2017.*

►♂**Quanah:** *Means "fragrant" in Comanche. This was the name of a 19th-century chief of the Comanche.*

**Pronunciation**: *KWAH-nə*

*The number of births with name Quanah is less than 5 of total male births in 2017.*

# LETTER R:

▶♀**Raisa:** Feminine form of Rais "leader, chief" in Arabic. Also "rose" in Yiddish

Pronunciation: ru-EES-ə

*The number of births with name Raisa is 22 of total female births in 2017.*

▶♂**Ralph:** From the Old Norse Rathulfr, composed of the elements rath (counsel) and ulfr (wolf). The name evolved into Rauf, Raff, and Rafe in the Middle Ages, Ralf in the 16th century, and Ralph in the 18th century.

Pronunciation: RALF – RAYF

*The number of births with name Ralph is 184 of total male births in 2017.*

▶♂**Raniel:** Meaning "God is my Joy" in Hebrew. Combination of the name Rani "my joy" or "my song" and El, reference to God. Other possible forms may be: Rhaniel, Rhanniel, Ranielle (female)

Pronunciation: RAYN-yəl

*The number of births with name Raniel is less than 5 of total male births in 2017.*

▶♀**Raphaela:** Feminine form of Raphael, from the Hebrew name רָפָאֵל (Rafa'el) which meant "God heals", from the roots אָ פָ ר (rafa') meaning "to heal" and לֵ א ('el) meaning "God".

**Pronunciation:** ra-fa-E-la

*The number of births with name Raphaela is 14 of total female births in 2017.*

▶♂**Raynar:** From the Germanic name Raganhar, composed of the elements ragin "advice" and hari "army".

Pronunciation: RAY-nər

*The number of births with name Raynar is 15 of total male births in 2017.*

▶♂**Ramsey:** Male name derived derived from the name Hræm's Island, which is from the Old English elements hræm(n) (raven) and ég, íg (island)

Pronunciation: RAM-zee

*The number of births with name Ramsey is 152 of total male births in 2017.*

▶♂**Rasmus:** Scandinavian, Finnish and Estonian form of Erasmus, derived from Greek ερασμιος (erasmios) meaning "beloved". Saint Erasmus, also known as Saint Elmo, was a 4th-century martyr who is the patron saint of sailors. Erasmus was also the name of a Dutch scholar of the Renaissance period.

**Pronunciation:** RAHS-moos

*The number of births with name Rasmus is less than 5 of total male births in 2017.*

▶♀**Rhonda:** Probably intended to mean "good spear" from Welsh rhon "spear" and da "good," but possibly influenced by the name of the Rhondda Valley in South Wales, which means "noisy." It has been in use only since the 20th century. Its use may have been partially inspired by Margaret Mackworth, Viscountess Rhondda (1883-1956), a British feminist.

Pronunciation: RAHN-də

*The number of births with name Ramsey is 19 of total female births in 2017.*

▶♀**Rhoda:** Derived from Greek "rose". As an English given name, Rhoda came into use in the 17th century.

**Pronunciation:** RO-də

*The number of births with name Rhoda is 41 of total female births in 2017.*

▶♀**Rosaline:** Derived from the Germanic elements hros meaning "horse" and lind meaning "soft, tender, flexible." The Normans introduced this name to England, though it was not common. During the Middle Ages, its spelling was influenced by the Latin phrase rosa linda "beautiful rose." The name was popularized by Edmund Spencer, who used it in his poetry, and by William Shakespeare, who used it for the heroine in his comedy 'As You Like It' (1599).

**Pronunciation:** ROZ-ə-l!nd

*The number of births with name Rosaline is 54 of total female births in 2017.*

►♂**Rudolf:** From the Germanic name Hrodulf, which was derived from the elements hrod "fame" and wulf "wolf."

**Pronunciation:** ROO-dolf

*The number of births with name Rudolf is 8 of total male births in 2017.*

►♀**Rue:** From the name of the bitter medicinal herb, ultimately deriving from Greek ῥυτη (rhyte).

**Pronunciation:** ROO

*The number of births with name Rue is 44 of total female births in 2017.*

*"ALWAYS END THE NAME OF YOUR CHILD WITH A VOWEL, SO THAT WHEN YOU YELL THE NAME WILL CARRY."*

BILL COSBY

# Chapter 4. **UNIQUE BABY NAMES S TO Z**

## **LETTER S:**

▶♀**Sabine:** French and German form of Sabina, which means "woman of the Sabine people", the Italian tribe from which, according to legend, the ancient Romans kidnapped their wives-to-be to populate their newly-founded city.

**Pronunciation:** sah-BEEN

*For 2017, the number of births with name Sabine is 94, which represents 0.0055 percent of total female births in 2017.*

▶♀**Saffron:** From the English word which refers either to the spice, the crocus flower from which it is harvested, or the yellow-orange color of the spice. It is ultimately derived from Arabic za'faran.

**Pronunciation:** SA-frawn

*For 2017, the number of births with name Saffron is 21, which represents 0.0012 percent of total female births in 2017.*

▶♀♂**Sage:** from the English word sage, which denotes either a type of spice or else a wise person.

**Pronunciation:** SAYJ

*For 2017, the number of births with name Sage is 1043, which represents 0.056 percent of total female births in 2017.*

*For 2017, the number of births with name Sage is 626, which represents 0.032 percent of total male births in 2017.*

▶ ♀**Sakura:** From Japanese 桜 "cherry blossom". It can also come from 咲 (saku) "blossom" and 良 (ra) "good."

**Pronunciation:** sah kuu rah

*For 2017, the number of births with name Sakura is 68, which represents 0.0064 percent of total female births in 2017.*

▶ ♀**Salma:** Means "safe", derived from Arabic salima "to be safe."

**Pronunciation:** SAHL-mah

*For 2017, the number of births with name Salma is 361, which represents 0.019 percent of total female births in 2017.*

▶ ♀**Salome:** From an Aramaic name which was related to the Hebrew word shalom meaning "peace". According to the historian Josephus, this was the name of the daughter of Herodias.

**Pronunciation:** SAHL-oh-may

*For 2017, the number of births with name Salome is 129, which represents 0.0075 percent of total female births in 2017.*

▶♀**Samara:** Possibly derived from the biblical place name Samaria, which means "watch mountain" in Hebrew

**Pronunciation:** sah-MAH-rə

*For 2017, the number of births with name Samara is 1002, which represents 0.053 percent of total female births in 2017.*

▶♂**Samson:** From the Hebrew name Shimshon which probably meant "sun". Samson was an Old Testament hero granted exceptional strength by God.

**Pronunciation:** SAM-sən

*For 2017, the number of births with name Samson is 430, which represents 0.022 percent of total male births in 2017.*

▶♀♂**Santana:** From the traditionally Spanish surname derived from any of the numerous places named Santa ANA.

**Pronunciation:** san-TA-nə

*For 2017, the number of births with name Santana is 236, which represents 0.0013 percent of total male births in 2017.*

*For 2017, the number of births with name Santana is 101, which represents 0.0059 percent of total female births in 2017.*

▶♂**Santino:** Diminutive of Santo, means "saint" in Italian, ultimately from Latin sanctus.

**Pronunciation:** sahn-TEE-noh

*For 2017, the number of births with name Santino is 444, which represents 0.023 percent of total male births in 2017.*

▶♂**Seamus:** Irish form of JAMES ("holder of the heel" or "supplanter").

**Pronunciation:** SHAY-məs

*For 2017, the number of births with name Seamus is 210, which represents 0.011 percent of total male births in 2017.*

▶♀**Sephora:** Greek form of Zipporah, from the Hebrew name צִפּוֹרָה (Tzipporah,) derived from צִפּוֹר (tzippor) meaning "bird".

**Pronounced:** zi-PAWR-ə

*For 2017, the number of births with name Sephora is 45, which represents 0.0026 percent of total female births in 2017.*

▶♀**Seraphina:** Feminine form of the Late Latin name Seraphinus, derived from the biblical word seraphim which were Hebrew in origin and meant "fiery ones." The seraphim were an order of angels. Seraphina was the name of a 13th-century Italian saint who made clothes for the poor.

**Pronunciation:** seh-rə-FEE-nə

*For 2017, the number of births with name Seraphina is 204, which represents 0.011 percent of total female births in 2017.*

▶♀♂**Shea:** Anglicized feminine form of Séaghdha, possibly means "admirable" or "hawk-like" in Gaelic.

**Pronounced:** SHAY

*For 2017, the number of births with name Shea is 182, which represents 0.011 percent of total female births in 2017.*

*For 2017, the number of births with name Shea is 125, which represents 0.0068 percent of total male births in 2017.*

▶♀♂**Shiloh:** From an Old Testament place name meaning "tranquil" in Hebrew. It is also used prophetically in the Old Testament to refer to a person, often understood to be the Messiah (see Genesis 49:10).

**Pronunciation:** SHIY-loh

*For 2017, the number of births with name Shiloh is 514, which represents 0.027 percent of total female births in 2017.*

*For 2017, the number of births with name Shiloh is 274, which represents 0.014 percent of total male births in 2017.*

▶♀**Sienna:** From the English word meaning "orange-red". It is ultimately from the name of the city of Siena in Italy, because of the color of the clay.

**Related to:** Sienna

**Pronunciation:** see-EH-nə

*For 2017, the number of births with name Siena is 454, which represents 0.024 percent of total female births in 2017.*

▶♂**Sirius:** The name of a bright star in the constellation Canis Major, derived via Latin from Greek σειριος (seirios) "burning".

**Pronounced:** SEER-ee-əs

*For 2017, the number of births with name Sirius is 38, which represents 0.0021 percent of total male births in 2017.*

▶♀♂**Sloane:** From an Irish surname which was derived from an Anglicized form of the given name Sluaghadhán.

**Pronounced:** SLON or SLOHN

*For 2017, the number of births with name Sloane is 1397, which represents 0.075 percent of total female births in 2017.*

*For 2017, the number of births with name Sloane is 8 in 2017.*

► ♀♂**Sunny:** From the English word meaning "sunny, cheerful."

**Pronounced:** SUN-ee

*For 2017, the number of births with name Sunny is 264, which represents 0.014 percent of total female births in 2017.*

*For 2017, the number of births with name Sunny is 59, which represents 0.032 percent of total male births in 2017.*

# LETTER T:

▶♂**Tadeo:** Spanish form of Thaddeus, from Θαδδαιος (Thaddaios), the Greek form of the Aramaic name Thaddai. It is possibly derived from a word meaning "heart," but it may, in fact, be an Aramaic form of a Greek name such as Θεοδωρος (see Theodore). In the Gospel of Matthew, Thaddaeus is listed as one of the twelve apostles.

Pronunciation: tə-DAY-oh

*For 2017, the number of births with name Tadeo is 264, which represents 0.014 percent of total male births in 2017.*

▶♀♂**Tate:** From an English surname which was derived from the Old English given name Tata of unknown origin

**Pronunciation:** TAYT

*For 2017, the number of births with name Tate is 677, which represents 0.034 percent of total male births in 2017.*

For 2017, the number of births with name Tate is 52, which represents 0.003 percent of total female births in 2017.

▶♀♂**Tatum:** From a surname which was originally derived from a place name meaning "Tata's homestead" in Old English

**Pronunciation:** TAY-təm

*For 2017, the number of births with name Tatum is 710, which represents 0.038 percent of total female births in 2017.*

*For 2017, the number of births with name Tatum is 449, which represents 0.023 percent of total male births in 2017.*

▶ ♀**Taya:** Japanese origin meaning "young."

**Pronounced:** TAH-yah or TIY-ə

For 2017, the number of births with name Taya is 195, which represents 0.011 percent of total female births in 2017.

▶ ♀**Temperance:** from the English word meaning "moderation" or "restraint."

**Pronunciation:** TEHM-per-ins

*For 2017, the number of births with name Temperance is 189, which represents 0.011 percent of total female births in 2017.*

▶ ♀**Thais:** Possibly means "bandage" in Greek

**Pronunciation:** tiy-EES

*For 2017, the number of births with name Thais is 26, which represents 0.0015 percent of total female births in 2017.*

► ♀**Thalia:** From the Greek Θαλεια (Thaleia), derived from θαλλω (thallo) meaning "to blossom". In Greek mythology, she was one of the nine Muses, the muse of comedy and pastoral poetry. This was also the name of one of the three Graces or Χαριτες (Charites).

**Pronunciation:** TAH-lee-ə, THAH-lee-ə

*For 2017, the number of births with name Thalia is 348, which represents 0.019 percent of total female births in 2017.*

► ♀**Thea:** Short form of Dorothea or Theodora ("gift of God").

**Pronunciation:** THEE-ə, THAY-ə, TAY-ə

*For 2017, the number of births with name Thea is 1180, which represents 0.063 percent of total female births in 2017.*

► ♂**Thelonious:** Anglicized form of Thelonius. Latinized form of Tielo, meaning 'ruler of the people'.

**Pronunciation:** theh-LOH-nee-əs

*For 2017, the number of births with name Thelonious is 23, which represents 0.0013 percent of total male births in 2017.*

► ♂**Thor:** From the Old Norse Þórr meaning "thunder", ultimately from the early Germanic *Þunraz.

Thor was the Norse god of strength, thunder, and war, the son of Odin.

**Pronunciation:** THOHR

*For 2017, the number of births with name Thor is 97, which represents 0.0053 percent of total male births in 2017.*

▶♂**Tiago:** Portuguese form of James derived from Santiago or "Saint James", derived from Spanish santo "saint" combined with Yago, an old Spanish form of James, the patron saint of Spain.

**Pronounced:** TEE-ah-goh or tchee-A-go

*For 2017, the number of births with name Tiago is 121, which represents 0.0066 percent of total male births in 2017.*

▶♂**Tobias:** Greek form of Tobiah orTōbias, which is from the Hebrew Tuviya, a name derived from tōbhīyāh (the Lord is good, God is good). This is the name of the hero of the apocryphal Book of Tobit in many English versions of the Old Testament.

**Pronunciation:** toh-BIY-əs

*For 2017, the number of births with name Tobias is 1320, which represents 0.067 percent of total male births in 2017.*

▶♀**Tyra:** From the Old Norse name Þýri, which was derived from the name of the Norse god Þórr (see Thor) combined with an unknown second element, possibly víg "war".

**Pronunciation:** TIY-rə

*For 2017, the number of births with name Tyra is 65, which represents 0.0038 percent of total female births in 2017.*

# LETTER U:

►♂**Ulrich:** From the Germanic name Odalric meaning "prosperity and power," from the element uodal "heritage" combined with ric "power."

**Pronounced as** OOL-rick

*For 2017, the number of births with name Ulrich is 10, which represents 0.0005 percent of total male births in 2017.*

►♀**Uma:** Means "flax" in Sanskrit. This is another name of the Hindu goddess Parvati.

**Pronunciation:** UU-mah

*For 2017, the number of births with name Uma is 73, which represents 0.0043 percent of total female births in 2017.*

►♀**Unity:** From the English word unity, which is ultimately derived from Latin unitas

**Pronunciation:** YOO-nə-tee

*For 2017, the number of births with name Unity is 30, which represents 0.0018 percent of total female births in 2017.*

►♂**Uriel:** From the Hebrew name 'Uri'el which meant "God is my light". Uriel was one of the seven archangels in Hebrew tradition.

**Pronunciation:** YUWR-ee-əl

*For 2017, the number of births with name Uriel is 537, which represents 0.027 percent of total male births in 2017.*

# LETTER V:

▶♀**Valentina:** Feminine form of Valentinus From the Roman cognomen Valentinus which was itself from the name Valens meaning "strong, vigorous, healthy" in Latin.

**Pronunciation:** va-lin-TEE-na

*For 2017, the number of births with name Valentina is 3027, which represents 0.161 percent of total female births in 2017.*

▶♂**Valentino:** See Valentina.

**Pronounced:** va-lin-TEE-no or va-len-TEE-no

*For 2017, the number of births with name Valentino is 375, which represents 0.019 percent of total male births in 2017.*

▶♀**Vega:** The name of a star in the constellation Lyra. Its name is from the Arabic al-Waqi' meaning "the swooping (eagle)". Vega Is THE brightest star in the summer sky.

**Pronunciation:** VAY-gə

*For 2017, the number of births with name Vega is 39, which represents 0.0033 percent of total female births in 2017.*

▶ ♀**Verena:** Possibly related to Latin verus "true". This might also be a Coptic form of the Ptolemaic name Berenice. Saint Verena was a 3rd-century Egyptian-born nurse.

**Pronounced:** ve-RE-na

*For 2017, the number of births with name Verena is 30, which represents 0.0018 percent of total female births in 2017.*

▶ ♀**Vienna:** From the name of the city in Austria, derived from Roman Vindobona, from Celtic vindo "white" and bona "foundation, fort". The "white" might be a reference to the river flowing through it. This name was borne by Vienna da Fuscaldo, mother of Saint Francis of Paola.

**Pronunciation:** vee-EH-nə

*For 2017, the number of births with name Vienna is 297, which represents 0.016 percent of total female births in 2017.*

▶ ♀**Vittoria:** Italian form of Victoria, the Feminine form of Victorius. Means "victory" in Latin. Victoria was the Roman goddess of victory.

**Pronounced:** vi-TAWR-ee-ə

*For 2017, the number of births with name Vittoria is 41, which represents 0.0024 percent of total female births in 2017.*

▶♂**Vladimir:** Means "to rule with greatness", derived from the Slavic element volod "rule" combined with mer "great, famous". The second element has also been associated with mir meaning "peace" or "world."

**Pronunciation:** vlah-DEE-meer

*For 2017, the number of births with name Vladimir is 161, which represents 0.0088 percent of total male births in 2017.*

# LETTER W:

▶ ♀**Waris:** Means "desert flower" in Somali.

**Pronunciation:** WAA-ris

*For 2017, the number of births with name Waris is 16, which represents 0.0017 percent of total female births in 2017.*

▶ ♀**Waverley or Waverly:** The name Waverly/Waverley is of Old English origin, meaning "quaking aspen."

**Pronunciation:** WAY-ver-lee

*For 2017, the number of births with name Waverley is 7, which represents 0.0004 percent of total female births in 2017.*

▶ ♂**Wilkes:** Diminutive of Will, from the Germanic name Willahelm, which was composed of the elements wil "will, desire" and helm "helmet, protection".

**Pronounced:** WIL-kes

*For 2017, the number of births with name Wilkes is 11, which represents 0.0006 percent of total male births in 2017.*

▶ ♀**Willa:** Feminine form of William, see Wilkes

**Pronunciation:** WI-lə

*For 2017, the number of births with name Willa is 691, which represents 0.037 percent of total female births in 2017.*

► ♀**Winona:** Means "firstborn daughter" in the Dakota/ Sioux language.

**Pronunciation:** wi-NOH-nə

*For 2017, the number of births with name Winona is 75, which represents 0.0044 percent of total female births in 2017.*

► ♀**Wren:** From the English word for the small songbird. It is ultimately derived from Old English wrenna or wroenna.

**Pronunciation:** REHN

*For 2017, the number of births with name Wren is 668, which represents 0.036 percent of total female births in 2017.*

# LETTER X:

▶♂**Xander:** Short form of Alexander ("defending men")

**Pronunciation:** ZAN-der

*For 2017, the number of births with name Xander is 2396, which represents 0.122 percent of total male births in 2017.*

*For 2017, the number of female births with name Xander is 7.*

▶♀**Ximena:** Feminine form of Ximeno, Medieval Spanish or Basque name of uncertain meaning, possibly a form of Simon, though it may in fact derive from Basque seme meaning "son".

**Pronunciation:** hee-MEH-nah, see-MEH-nah

*For 2017, the number of births with name Ximena is 2534, which represents 0.135 percent of total female births in 2017.*

▶♀**Xiomara:** Possibly a Spanish form of Guiomar, possibly derived from the Germanic name Wigmar meaning "famous in war."

**Pronunciation:** soo-oh-MAH-rah

*For 2017, the number of births with name Xiomara is 319, which represents 0.017 percent of total female births in 2017.*

▶ ♀**Xoey:** Variant of Zoe, Means "life" in Greek.

**Pronounced:** ZO-eei

*For 2017, the number of births with name Xoey is 13, which represents 0.0007 percent of total female births in 2017.*

▶ ♀**Xylia:** Modern creation, perhaps based on Greek ξυλον (xylon) meaning "of the forest."

Pronounced: ZYE-lee-uh

*For 2017, the number of births with name Xylia is 17, which represents 0.0009 percent of total female births in 2017.*

# LETTER Y:

▶♂**Yael:** Hebrew form of JAEL, from the Hebrew name יָעֵל (Ya'el) meaning "ibex, mountain goat".

**Pronunciation:** yah-EHL

*For 2017, the number of births with name Yael is 197, which represents 0.011 percent of total male births in 2017.*

▶♀**Yasmin:** From Persian ياسمن (yasamen) meaning "jasmine."

**Pronunciation:** yahz-MEEN

*For 2017, the number of births with name Yasmin is 251, which represents 0.015 percent of total female births in 2017.*

▶♀**Yuliana:** Russian and Bulgarian form of Juliana. Feminine form of Iulianus (see Julianne).

**Pronunciation:** Ew-lih-AH-nah

*For 2017, the number of births with name Yuliana is 170, which represents 0.0099 percent of total female births in 2017.*

▶♂**Yves:** Medieval French form of Ivo. This was the name of two French saints: an 11th-century bishop of Chartres and a 13th-century parish priest and lawyer, also known as Ivo of Kermartin, the patron saint of Brittany.

**Pronunciation:** EEV

*For 2017, the number of births with name Yves is 22, which represents 0.0012 percent of total male births in 2017.*

# LETTER Z:

▶♂**Zac:** Short form of Zachary, the Greek form of Zechariah. This form of the name is used in most English versions of the New Testament to refer to the father of John the Baptist.

**Related to:** Zacharias or Zachary

*For 2017, the number of births with name Xac is 67, which represents 0.0037 percent of total male births in 2017.*

▶♀**Zafira:** Variant transcription of Sapphira. From the Greek name Σαπφειρη (Sappheire), which was from Greek σαπφειρος (sappheiros) meaning "sapphire" or "lapis lazuli" (ultimately derived from the Hebrew word סַפִּיר (sappir)).

**Pronunciation:** zah-FEE-rə

*For 2017, the number of births with name Zafira is 13, which represents 0.0007 percent of total female births in 2017.*

▶♀**Zaida:** Feminine form of Zayd, derived from Arabic zada "to increase".

**Pronunciation:** ZAY-də

For 2017, the number of births with name Zaida is 89, which represents 0.0052 percent of total female births in 2017.

► ♀**Zain:** Variant transcription of Zayn, means "beauty, grace" in Arabic

**Pronunciation:** ZAYN

*For 2017, the number of births with name Zain is 399, which represents 0.020 percent of total male births in 2017.*

*For 2017, the number of births with name Zain is 10, which represents 0.00005 percent of total female births in 2017.*

► ♀**Zara:** English form of ZAÏRE. In England, it came to public attention when Princess Anne gave it to her daughter in 1981. The trendy Spanish clothing retailer Zara may also influence use of the name.

**Pronounced:** ZAHR-ə

*For 2017, the number of births with name Zara is 1149, which represents 0.061 percent of total female births in 2017.*

► ♀**Zelda:** Of uncertain etymology, Zelda is thought by some to be a variant spelling of Selda, a name from the Old English selda (companion). Alternatively, Zelda is a Yiddish cognate of the German Salida (happiness, joy). May also be a short form of Griselda or used because of a popular video game.

**Pronunciation:** ZEHL-də

*For 2017, the number of births with name Zelda is 454, which represents 0.024 percent of total female births in 2017.*

▶♂**Zephyr:** From the Greek Ζεφυρος (Zephyros) meaning "the west wind". Zephyros was the Greek god of the west wind.

**Pronounced:** ZEF-ər

*For 2017, the number of births with name Zephyr is 127, which represents 0.0069 percent of total male births in 2017.*

*"TIGERS DIE AND LEAVE THEIR SKINS; PEOPLE DIE AND LEAVE THEIR NAMES."*

JAPANESE PROVERB

# CHAPTER 5: KEY TO PRONUNCIATION.

This book uses two systems for name pronunciations: basic, which is a rough guide, and IPA, which is more exact. The /slashes/ surrounding they can identify IPA (International Phonetic Alphabet) pronunciations.

Dashes are used to separate syllables. Stressed syllables are written in **CAPITALS**.

## VOWEL SOUNDS

| Written | Sound |
|---------|-------|
| a | a as in cat |
| ah | a as in father or o as in on |
| aw | aw as in dawn |
| ay | a as in ate or é as in café |
| er | er as in farmer |
| ə | a neutral, unstressed vowel as in sofa or upon |
| ee | e as in here |
| eh | e as in pet |
| i | i as in sit |
| iy | i as in bite or y as in my |
| oh | o as in tone |
| oo | oo as boot or u as in flute |
| ow | ow as in brown |
| oy | oy as in boy |
| uh | u as in fun |
| uw | u as in put or oo as in wood |

## AMBIGUOUS CONSONANT SOUNDS

| Written | Sound |
|---------|-------|
| ch | ch as in choose |
| g | g as in gate |
| j | j as in jump or g as in giant |
| kh | unvoiced throat sounds that soften to an "h" in English, like jalapeño and Chaim |
| ng | ng as in walking or n as in anchor |
| s | s as in soft or c as in race |
| z | z as in zebra or s as in jeans |
| th | unvoiced th as in thin |
| dh | voiced th as in there |
| zh | s as in measure or t as in equation |

See IPA reference here:

https://en.wikipedia.org/wiki/International_Phonetic_Alphabet

# Gender Symbols:

♀ → It's usually used as a Female name.

♂ → It's usually used as a Male name.

*"THE NAME OF A MAN IS A NUMBING BLOW FROM WHICH HE NEVER RECOVERS."*

MARSHALL MCLUHAN

# CHAPTER 6: TIPS FOR CHOOSING A NAME.

**Think of your child's future:** Choose the name for your baby's benefit, NOT yours. This means no joke names, puns or plays on words. Don´t Name your baby to tell the world all about you.

**Know what you are looking for:** Are you thinking of a traditional, religious or an uncommon name? Would you like a short or long name? This will help to narrow down your search.

**How does it sound like?** How does the name sound with your surname? Think about your baby's name. Say it aloud. Does it have a melody? Do you think it sounds weird or out of place? Avoid choosing a name that rhymes with or is too similar to your surname.

**Ancestry and heritage:** Your child's heritage is very important, and you may want their name to show it.

**Initials and nicknames:** Check your baby's initials don't spell out an unfortunate word. Do you like the shortened version of the name?

**Celebrity:** You may be planning to name your baby after a celebrity (Real or Fictional) with an unusual name, think how it will sound in 40 years.

**Keep it secret:** try to keep the baby's name a secret between you and your spouse until the baby's born. You may not appreciate another people's opinion.

**Does the name go with the names of your older children?** Try not to choose names that are too like those you chose for older siblings.

**Can you imagine your baby as an adult with this name?** Bear in mind that your baby will become an adult one day. Pick Names that age well.

**Will other people be able to spell your baby's name?** An unusual pronunciation of a name can cause endless confusion. You and your child will soon grow tired of correcting people when they misspell her name or can't pronounce it.

**Do you both love the name?** If choosing a name is hard for one parent, finding something you both like is even trickier. But if your partner hates your favorite name, don't force it.

**Is it a Popular Pet Name?** You don't want your baby named like the neighbor's dog.

**Is It Overly Popular?** You may not want your son to be named like 10 of his friends.

**Will You Still Love It Tomorrow?** Test if for a few days, say it loud, if you don't like it the next day, change it.

**Bypass A Family Name:** It's always a nice tribute to name a child after a beloved grandma or grandpop, but even though some old-fashioned names are back in a big way.

**Wait Until You Meet Him or her:** It might sound like the ultimate in procrastination but taking the wait-and-see approach makes sense for some couples.

**Spell it clearly**. A unique spelling can seem like a way to make a common name stand out, but you may not love continually correcting people, imagine your baby doing it all his life.

**Uniqueness:** sometimes an extremely unusual name can bring your child unwanted attention instead.

**Consider using a middle name**, sometimes may help to solve naming problems or to make everyone happy.

# BONUS MATERIAL: How Popular is a name?

## TOP 1000 NAMES IN THE U.S.

| | Name | S | Meaning | Origin | Births |
|---|---|---|---|---|---|
| 1 | Emma | F | Very Industrious | German | 19738 |
| 2 | Liam | M | Resolute protector | Irish | 18728 |
| 3 | Olivia | F | From Olive tree | Latin | 18632 |
| 4 | Noah | M | Rest or comfort | Hebrew | 18326 |
| 5 | Ava | F | Like a bird | Latin | 15902 |
| 6 | Isabella | F | Consecrated to God | Italian | 15100 |
| 7 | William | M | Resolute protector | German | 14904 |
| 8 | Sophia | F | Wisdom | Greek | 14831 |
| 9 | James | M | Supplanted | English | 14232 |
| 10 | Logan | M | Dweller in a little hollow | Irish | 13974 |
| 11 | Benjamin | M | Born of the right hand | Hebrew | 13733 |
| 12 | Mason | M | Stoneworker | French | 13502 |
| 13 | Mia | F | Wished for child | Hebrew | 13437 |
| 14 | Elijah | M | The Lord is my God | Hebrew | 13268 |
| 15 | Oliver | M | Olive tree | Latin | 13141 |
| 16 | Jacob | M | Supplanted | Hebrew | 13106 |
| 17 | Lucas | M | Bringer of light | Latin | 12951 |
| 18 | Charlotte | F | Little and womanly | French | 12893 |
| 19 | Michael | M | Who is like God | Hebrew | 12579 |
| 20 | Alexander | M | Defender of mankind | Greek | 12467 |
| 21 | Ethan | M | Strength or long-lived | Hebrew | 12389 |
| 22 | Amelia | F | Very Industrious | Latin | 11800 |
| 23 | Daniel | M | God is my judge | Hebrew | 11640 |
| 24 | Matthew | M | A Gift from God | Hebrew | 11611 |
| 25 | Aiden | M | Little fiery one | Irish | 11259 |
| 26 | Evelyn | F | Hazelnut | Old English | 10675 |
| 27 | Abigail | F | Rejoice of My father | Hebrew | 10551 |
| 28 | Harper | F | Harpist or minstrel | English | 10451 |
| 29 | Henry | M | Ruler of the enclosure | German | 10406 |

| 30 | Joseph | M | God will add | Hebrew | 10360 |
|---|---|---|---|---|---|
| 31 | Jackson | M | God is gracious | Old English | 10356 |
| 32 | Samuel | M | Heard by God | Hebrew | 10323 |
| 33 | Sebastian | M | Venerable, revered | Latin | 10136 |
| 34 | David | M | Beloved | Hebrew | 10124 |
| 35 | Carter | M | Transporter of goods with a cart | Old English | 9753 |
| 36 | Emily | F | Industrious | German | 9746 |
| 37 | Wyatt | M | To lead | English | 9661 |
| 38 | Jayden | M | Jade | American | 9495 |
| 39 | John | M | God is gracious | Hebrew | 9434 |
| 40 | Owen | M | Wellborn | Welsh | 9312 |
| 41 | Dylan | M | Son of the sea | Welsh | 9268 |
| 42 | Luke | M | Bringer of light | Latin | 9163 |
| 43 | Gabriel | M | God is my strength | Hebrew | 9083 |
| 44 | Elizabeth | F | God is my oath | Hebrew | 8915 |
| 45 | Anthony | M | Priceless, inestimable or praiseworthy | Latin | 8802 |
| 46 | Isaac | M | Laughter | Hebrew | 8796 |
| 47 | Grayson | M | Son of the gray-haired man | Old English | 8640 |
| 48 | Jack | M | God is gracious | Old English | 8419 |
| 49 | Julian | M | Downy bearded or youthful | Latin | 8393 |
| 50 | Levi | M | Joined or united | Hebrew | 8367 |
| 51 | Christopher | M | Christ-bearer | Greek | 8255 |
| 52 | Joshua | M | God is salvation | Hebrew | 8239 |
| 53 | Andrew | M | Manly | Greek | 8215 |
| 54 | Avery | F | Elf ruler | English | 8186 |
| 55 | Lincoln | M | Settlement by the pool | Old English | 8146 |
| 56 | Sofia | F | Wisdom | Greek | 8134 |
| 57 | Ella | F | Foreign | French | 8014 |
| 58 | Madison | F | Mighty in battle | English | 7847 |
| 59 | Mateo | M | Gift of God | Spanish | 7726 |
| 60 | Scarlett | F | Bright red | English | 7679 |
| 61 | Ryan | M | Little King | Irish | 7652 |
| 62 | Jaxon | M | God has been gracious | American | 7649 |
| 63 | Nathan | M | Gift from God | Hebrew | 7390 |
| 64 | Victoria | F | Victory | Latin | 7267 |

| 65 | Aaron | M | Exalted one | Hebrew | 7165 |
|---|---|---|---|---|---|
| 66 | Isaiah | M | God is my salvation | Hebrew | 7165 |
| 67 | Aria | F | Gentle music | Greek | 7132 |
| 68 | Thomas | M | Twin | Greek | 7131 |
| 69 | Charles | M | Manly | English | 7130 |
| 70 | Caleb | M | Faithful dog | Hebrew | 7084 |
| 71 | Grace | F | Beauty of form | Latin | 6991 |
| 72 | Josiah | M | Jehovah has healed | Hebrew | 6976 |
| 73 | Christian | M | Follower of Christ or anointed | Greek | 6968 |
| 74 | Chloe | F | Blooming | Greek | 6912 |
| 75 | Camila | F | Young ceremonial attendant | Spanish | 6752 |
| 76 | Hunter | M | A huntsman | English | 6701 |
| 77 | Penelope | F | Weaver | Greek | 6639 |
| 78 | Eli | M | Uplifted or ascent | Hebrew | 6553 |
| 79 | Jonathan | M | Gift of God | Hebrew | 6471 |
| 80 | Connor | M | Exalted | Irish | 6382 |
| 81 | Riley | F | Dweller by the rye field | Old English | 6343 |
| 82 | Landon | M | Open grassy meadow | Old English | 6326 |
| 83 | Layla | F | Wine | Arabic | 6274 |
| 84 | Adrian | M | Dark | Latin | 6203 |
| 85 | Lillian | F | Lily | Latin | 6132 |
| 86 | Nora | F | Bright Torch | Greek | 6036 |
| 87 | Zoey | F | Life | Greek | 6026 |
| 88 | Asher | M | Blessed | Hebrew | 5991 |
| 89 | Mila | F | Loved by the people | Slavic | 5941 |
| 90 | Cameron | M | Crooked Nose | Scottish | 5925 |
| 91 | Leo | M | Lion | Latin | 5923 |
| 92 | Theodore | M | God's gift | Latin | 5911 |
| 93 | Aubrey | F | Blond ruler | French | 5891 |
| 94 | Hannah | F | Gracious | Hebrew | 5872 |
| 95 | Lily | F | Lily | Latin | 5816 |
| 96 | Jeremiah | M | God will uplift | Hebrew | 5815 |
| 97 | Hudson | M | Hugh's son | Old English | 5755 |
| 98 | Addison | F | Son of Adam | English | 5593 |
| 99 | Eleanor | F | Light | Greek | 5519 |
| 100 | Natalie | F | Born at Christmas | Latin | 5516 |

| 101 | Robert | M | Bright with fame | English | 5507 |
|---|---|---|---|---|---|
| 102 | Easton | M | Eastern settlement | Old English | 5486 |
| 103 | Nolan | M | Noble | Irish | 5375 |
| 104 | Nicholas | M | The victory of the people | Greek | 5321 |
| 105 | Luna | F | Moon | Spanish | 5320 |
| 106 | Ezra | M | Helper | Hebrew | 5290 |
| 107 | Colton | M | Coal town | Old English | 5253 |
| 108 | Angel | M | Messenger | Latin | 5240 |
| 109 | Savannah | F | A treeless place | Spanish | 5222 |
| 110 | Brooklyn | F | Stream by the lake | English | 5168 |
| 111 | Leah | F | Tired or weary | Hebrew | 5159 |
| 112 | Brayden | M | Broad valley | Old English | 5138 |
| 113 | Zoe | F | Life | Greek | 5129 |
| 114 | Jordan | M | To flow down or descend | Hebrew | 5114 |
| 115 | Dominic | M | Belonging to the lord | Latin | 5076 |
| 116 | Stella | F | Star | Latin | 5038 |
| 117 | Austin | M | Majestic | Latin | 5024 |
| 118 | Hazel | F | Hazelnut | Old English | 5004 |
| 119 | Ian | M | God is gracious | Scottish | 5002 |
| 120 | Ellie | F | Light | Greek | 4993 |
| 121 | Paisley | F | A Church | Scotish | 4927 |
| 122 | Adam | M | Red Earth | Hebrew | 4904 |
| 123 | Elias | M | Jehovah is God | Greek | 4894 |
| 124 | Jaxson | M | Son of Jack | Old English | 4820 |
| 125 | Greyson | M | Gray haired | English | 4819 |
| 126 | Audrey | F | Noble strength | Old English | 4808 |
| 127 | Jose | M | God will add | Spanish | 4775 |
| 128 | Ezekiel | M | Strength of God | Hebrew | 4721 |
| 129 | Carson | M | Marsh or mossy place | Scottish | 4718 |
| 130 | Evan | M | Youth warrior | Irish | 4709 |
| 131 | Skylar | F | The isle of Skye | Scottish | 4706 |
| 132 | Maverick | M | Unbranded | American | 4702 |
| 133 | Violet | F | Bluish purple | Latin | 4699 |
| 134 | Claire | F | Bright or clear | French | 4683 |
| 135 | Bryson | M | Son of the strong one | Welsh | 4633 |
| 136 | Jace | M | To heal | Greek | 4621 |

| 137 | Bella | F | Beautiful | Latin | 4611 |
|-----|-------|---|-----------|-------|------|
| 138 | Cooper | M | A barrel maker or seller | English | 4581 |
| 139 | Aurora | F | Dawn | Latin | 4573 |
| 140 | Lucy | F | Bringer of light | Latin | 4564 |
| 141 | Anna | F | Grace | English | 4520 |
| 142 | Xavier | M | Owner of a new home | Basque | 4468 |
| 143 | Parker | M | Gamekeeper | English | 4346 |
| 144 | Samantha | F | Told by God | Hebrew | 4303 |
| 145 | Caroline | F | Little and womanly | French | 4270 |
| 146 | Roman | M | Roman | Latin | 4253 |
| 147 | Genesis | F | Beginning | Latin | 4241 |
| 148 | Jason | M | Healer | Greek | 4221 |
| 149 | Santiago | M | Supplanted | Spanish | 4188 |
| 150 | Aaliyah | F | Rising | Hebrew | 4160 |
| 151 | Chase | M | Huntsman | French | 4157 |
| 152 | Sawyer | M | Wood cutter | English | 4146 |
| 153 | Kennedy | F | Ugly head | Irish | 4137 |
| 154 | Gavin | M | White falcon | Welsh | 4134 |
| 155 | Leonardo | M | Brave as a lion | Italian/Spanish | 4113 |
| 156 | Kinsley | F | King's Meadow | Old English | 4035 |
| 157 | Allison | F | Truthful | Old English | 4017 |
| 158 | Maya | F | Industrious | Latin | 4008 |
| 159 | Sarah | F | Princess | Hebrew | 3986 |
| 160 | Kayden | M | | | 3969 |
| 161 | Madelyn | F | | | 3939 |
| 162 | Ayden | M | | | 3931 |
| 163 | Jameson | M | Supplanted | English | 3907 |
| 164 | Adeline | F | Noble | English | 3902 |
| 165 | Alexa | F | Defender of mankind | Greek | 3883 |
| 166 | Ariana | F | Holy | Greek | 3865 |
| 167 | Elena | F | Light | Greek | 3863 |
| 168 | Gabriella | F | God is my strength | Italian | 3862 |
| 169 | Naomi | F | Beautiful | Hebrew | 3823 |
| 170 | Kevin | M | Little gentle one or handsome | Irish | 3805 |
| 171 | Alice | F | Truthful | Greek | 3804 |
| 172 | Bentley | M | Bent grass | English | 3796 |

| | | | | | |
|---|---|---|---|---|---|
| 173 | Zachary | M | God remembers | Hebrew | 3779 |
| 174 | Everett | M | Strong as a wild boar | Scandinavian | 3766 |
| 175 | Axel | M | Father of peace | Scandinavian | 3764 |
| 176 | Tyler | M | Tile maker | French | 3744 |
| 177 | Sadie | F | Princess | Hebrew | 3695 |
| 178 | Hailey | F | From the hay meadow | English | 3691 |
| 179 | Micah | M | Who is like God | Hebrew | 3660 |
| 180 | Vincent | M | Conquering | Latin | 3651 |
| 181 | Weston | M | Town facing west | Old English | 3637 |
| 182 | Eva | F | Life | Hebrew | 3614 |
| 183 | Miles | M | Merciful | German | 3601 |
| 184 | Emilia | F | Industrious | Italian | 3581 |
| 185 | Autumn | F | Mature | Latin | 3575 |
| 186 | Quinn | F | Queen | Old English | 3575 |
| 187 | Nevaeh | F | | | 3562 |
| 188 | Wesley | M | A clearing in the west | Old English | 3547 |
| 189 | Piper | F | Piper | English | 3542 |
| 190 | Ruby | F | Reddish | Latin | 3540 |
| 191 | Serenity | F | Tranquility | Latin | 3537 |
| 192 | Willow | F | Graceful or slender | English | 3529 |
| 193 | Everly | F | From Ever's meadow | English | 3505 |
| 194 | Nathaniel | M | Gift of God | Latin | 3504 |
| 195 | Harrison | M | Son of Harry | Old English | 3499 |
| 196 | Brandon | M | Beacon hill | Old English | 3474 |
| 197 | Cole | M | Darkly complexioned | Old English | 3446 |
| 198 | Declan | M | Man of prayer | Irish | 3444 |
| 199 | Cora | F | Maiden | Greek | 3422 |
| 200 | Kaylee | F | Pure | American | 3390 |
| 201 | Luis | M | Famous warrior | Spanish | 3374 |
| 202 | Braxton | M | Brock's town | Old English | 3320 |
| 203 | Damian | M | To tame | Greek | 3316 |
| 204 | Lydia | F | Woman from Lydia | Greek | 3311 |
| 205 | Aubree | F | Blond ruler | French | 3302 |
| 206 | Silas | M | From the forest or woods | Latin | 3296 |
| 207 | Tristan | M | Bold | Welsh | 3285 |
| 208 | Arianna | F | | | 3264 |

| 209 | Eliana | F | God has answered me | Hebrew | 3254 |
|-----|--------|---|---------------------|--------|------|
| 210 | Peyton | F | Warrior's town | Old English | 3244 |
| 211 | Ryder | M | Knight | English | 3238 |
| 212 | Melanie | F | Dark skinned | Greek | 3227 |
| 213 | Gianna | F | God is gracious | Italian | 3183 |
| 214 | Bennett | M | Blessed | Latin | 3167 |
| 215 | George | M | Farmer | Greek | 3151 |
| 216 | Emmett | M | Industrious | German | 3145 |
| 217 | Isabelle | F | Consecrated to God | German | 3145 |
| 218 | Justin | M | Just | Latin | 3121 |
| 219 | Kai | M | Earth | Greek | 3121 |
| 220 | Max | M | By the great stream | Scottish | 3121 |
| 221 | Julia | F | Downy bearded or youthful | Latin | 3111 |
| 222 | Diego | M | Supplanted | Spanish | 3088 |
| 223 | Luca | M | Bringer of light | Italian | 3070 |
| 224 | Ryker | M | | | 3063 |
| 225 | Carlos | M | Manly | Spanish | 3058 |
| 226 | Maxwell | M | Dweller by the spring | Scottish | 3052 |
| 227 | Kingston | M | From the king's village or estate | Old English | 3038 |
| 228 | Ivan | M | God is gracious | Russian | 3031 |
| 229 | Valentina | F | Healthy or strong | Latin | 3027 |
| 230 | Nova | F | Chases butterfly | Hopi | 3026 |
| 231 | Clara | F | Bright or clear | Latin | 3022 |
| 232 | Maddox | M | Benefactor's son | Welsh | 3017 |
| 233 | Vivian | F | Full of life, lively or alive | French | 3013 |
| 234 | Reagan | F | Little king | Irish | 2999 |
| 235 | Juan | M | God is gracious | Spanish | 2980 |
| 236 | Mackenzie | F | | | 2941 |
| 237 | Madeline | F | From the high tower | Greek | 2938 |
| 238 | Ashton | M | Ash tree enclosure | Old English | 2937 |
| 239 | Jayce | M | | | 2885 |
| 240 | Brielle | F | Cheese | French | 2880 |
| 241 | Delilah | F | Delicate | Hebrew | 2873 |
| 242 | Isla | F | Isla river in Scotland | Scottish | 2863 |
| 243 | Rylee | F | Island meadow | Irish | 2847 |
| 244 | Katherine | F | Pure | Greek | 2833 |

| 245 | Rowan | M | From the rowan tree | English | 2827 |
| 246 | Sophie | F | | | 2820 |
| 247 | Kaiden | M | | | 2800 |
| 248 | Josephine | F | God will add | French | 2791 |
| 249 | Giovanni | M | God is gracious | Italian | 2783 |
| 250 | Eric | M | Eternal ruler | Scandinavian | 2757 |
| 251 | Ivy | F | Climber | Old English | 2756 |
| 252 | Liliana | F | Lily | Latin | 2747 |
| 253 | Jesus | M | Jehovah is salvation | Hebrew | 2735 |
| 254 | Jade | F | Stone of the side | Spanish | 2725 |
| 255 | Maria | F | Bitter or sea of bitterness | Hebrew | 2699 |
| 256 | Taylor | F | To cut | French | 2692 |
| 257 | Hadley | F | From the heather covered meadow | Old English | 2691 |
| 258 | Calvin | M | Bald | French | 2689 |
| 259 | Kylie | F | Beautiful | Irish | 2688 |
| 260 | Abel | M | Breath | Hebrew | 2686 |
| 261 | Emery | F | Industrious ruler | German | 2682 |
| 262 | King | M | Monarch | Old English | 2661 |
| 263 | Adalynn | F | | | 2651 |
| 264 | Camden | M | From the winding valley | Scottish | 2651 |
| 265 | Natalia | F | Born at Christmas | Latin | 2602 |
| 266 | Annabelle | F | | | 2601 |
| 267 | Amir | M | Prince | Arabic | 2600 |
| 268 | Blake | M | Dark complexioned | Old English | 2600 |
| 269 | Faith | F | Trust or belief | English | 2597 |
| 270 | Alexandra | F | Defender of mankind | Greek | 2592 |
| 271 | Alex | M | Defender of mankind | Greek | 2578 |
| 272 | Brody | M | A ditch | Irish | 2542 |
| 273 | Ximena | F | | | 2534 |
| 274 | Ashley | F | Meadow of ash trees | Old English | 2517 |
| 275 | Malachi | M | Messenger of God | Hebrew | 2507 |
| 276 | Brianna | F | Strong | Irish | 2504 |
| 277 | Emmanuel | M | God is with us | Hebrew | 2502 |
| 278 | Jonah | M | Dove | Hebrew | 2500 |
| 279 | Beau | M | Handsome or pretty | French | 2493 |
| 280 | Jude | M | Praised | Hebrew | 2493 |

| 281 | Antonio | M | Priceless, inestimable or praiseworthy | Italian | 2470 |
|---|---|---|---|---|---|
| 282 | Raelynn | F | | | 2437 |
| 283 | Alan | M | Handsome | Irish | 2436 |
| 284 | Elliott | M | Jehovah is God | French | 2421 |
| 285 | Bailey | F | Law enforcer or bailiff | Old English | 2420 |
| 286 | Elliot | M | Jehovah is God | French | 2416 |
| 287 | Waylon | M | From the land by the road | English | 2416 |
| 288 | Xander | M | | | 2396 |
| 289 | Timothy | M | One who honors God | Greek | 2393 |
| 290 | Victor | M | Conqueror | Latin | 2392 |
| 291 | Mary | F | Sea of bitterness | Hebrew | 2381 |
| 292 | Bryce | M | Strength or valor | Welsh | 2380 |
| 293 | Athena | F | Skill or wisdom | Greek | 2365 |
| 294 | Finn | M | Light skinned or blond | Irish | 2365 |
| 295 | Brantley | M | Proud | Old English | 2320 |
| 296 | Andrea | F | Manly | Greek | 2312 |
| 297 | Edward | M | Wealthy guardian | Old English | 2309 |
| 298 | Abraham | M | Father of a multitude | Hebrew | 2300 |
| 299 | Patrick | M | Nobleman | Latin | 2283 |
| 300 | Grant | M | Great plains | English | 2279 |
| 301 | Karter | M | | | 2273 |
| 302 | Hayden | M | From the hedged valley | English | 2272 |
| 303 | Richard | M | Rich and powerful ruler | English | 2269 |
| 304 | Miguel | M | Who is like God | Spanish | 2266 |
| 305 | Leilani | F | Heavenly flower | Hawaiian | 2264 |
| 306 | Jasmine | F | Fragrant flower | Arabic | 2256 |
| 307 | Lyla | F | From the island | French | 2251 |
| 308 | Joel | M | God is willing | Hebrew | 2242 |
| 309 | Margaret | F | Pearl | Greek | 2242 |
| 310 | Gael | M | My father rejoices | Hebrew | 2234 |
| 311 | Alyssa | F | Truthful | Greek | 2227 |
| 312 | Tucker | M | Garment maker | Old English | 2211 |
| 313 | Adalyn | F | Noble | English | 2194 |
| 314 | Rhett | M | Enthusiastic | Welsh | 2188 |
| 315 | Avery | M | Elf ruler | English | 2179 |
| 316 | Arya | F | | | 2156 |

| 317 | Norah | F | Light | Greek | 2148 |
|-----|-------|---|-------|-------|------|
| 318 | Steven | M | Crown or wreath | Latin | 2148 |
| 319 | Khloe | F | | | 2143 |
| 320 | Kayla | F | Pure | Greek | 2108 |
| 321 | Graham | M | Grand home | English | 2101 |
| 322 | Kaleb | M | Faithfulness | Hebrew | 2091 |
| 323 | Jasper | M | Treasurer | French | 2083 |
| 324 | Eden | F | Delight | Hebrew | 2082 |
| 325 | Jesse | M | Wealthy | Hebrew | 2074 |
| 326 | Matteo | M | Gift from God | Spanish | 2071 |
| 327 | Dean | M | Hollow or valley | Old English | 2067 |
| 328 | Eliza | F | God is my oath | Hebrew | 2061 |
| 329 | Rose | F | Flower | Latin | 2059 |
| 330 | Ariel | F | Lion of God | Hebrew | 2056 |
| 331 | Zayden | M | | | 2056 |
| 332 | Preston | M | The priest's village | Old English | 2055 |
| 333 | Melody | F | Melody or song | Greek | 2046 |
| 334 | Alexis | F | Defender of mankind | Greek | 2044 |
| 335 | August | M | Venerable | Latin | 2041 |
| 336 | Oscar | M | God's spear | Scandinavian | 2040 |
| 337 | Jeremy | M | God will uplift | English | 2035 |
| 338 | Alejandro | M | Defender of mankind | Spanish | 2027 |
| 339 | Isabel | F | Consecrated to God | Spanish | 2016 |
| 340 | Marcus | M | Warlike | Latin | 2011 |
| 341 | Sydney | F | Wide meadow | French | 2007 |
| 342 | Dawson | M | Beloved | English | 2004 |
| 343 | Lorenzo | M | Crowned with laurels | Italian | 1994 |
| 344 | Juliana | F | Downy bearded or youthful | Latin | 1991 |
| 345 | Lauren | F | Crowned with laurels | English | 1978 |
| 346 | Messiah | M | | | 1970 |
| 347 | Iris | F | Rainbow | Greek | 1969 |
| 348 | Emerson | F | Industrious ruler | German | 1965 |
| 349 | London | F | Fortress | Old English | 1957 |
| 350 | Zion | M | Sign | Hebrew | 1956 |
| 351 | Maximus | M | The greatest | Latin | 1951 |
| 352 | River | M | Flowing water | French | 1948 |

| 353 | Zane | M | God is Gracious | English | 1938 |
|---|---|---|---|---|---|
| 354 | Mark | M | Warlike | Latin | 1936 |
| 355 | Brooks | M | Son of Brooke | Old English | 1921 |
| 356 | Morgan | F | Bright Sea | Welsh | 1911 |
| 357 | Lilly | F | Lily | Latin | 1906 |
| 358 | Nicolas | M | Victory of the people | Greek | 1906 |
| 359 | Charlie | F | Manly | English | 1900 |
| 360 | Paxton | M | Peaceful town | Latin | 1898 |
| 361 | Aliyah | F | | | 1897 |
| 362 | Judah | M | Praised | Hebrew | 1897 |
| 363 | Valeria | F | To be strong | Latin | 1887 |
| 364 | Arabella | F | Beautiful alter | Latin | 1875 |
| 365 | Sara | F | Princess | Hebrew | 1872 |
| 366 | Emiliano | M | | | 1864 |
| 367 | Finley | F | | | 1859 |
| 368 | Trinity | F | Triad | Latin | 1846 |
| 369 | Ryleigh | F | Island meadow | Irish | 1845 |
| 370 | Kaden | M | Companion | Arabic | 1840 |
| 371 | Jordyn | F | | | 1829 |
| 372 | Jocelyn | F | Joyous | Latin | 1828 |
| 373 | Bryan | M | Honorable | Irish | 1827 |
| 374 | Kimberly | F | Fortress meadow | Old English | 1823 |
| 375 | Kyle | M | Land where cattle graze | Scottish | 1823 |
| 376 | Esther | F | Star | Arabic | 1820 |
| 377 | Molly | F | Bitter | Irish | 1819 |
| 378 | Valerie | F | To be strong | Latin | 1814 |
| 379 | Cecilia | F | Dim sighted or blind | Latin | 1804 |
| 380 | Myles | M | Merciful | German | 1792 |
| 381 | Anastasia | F | Resurrection | Greek | 1790 |
| 382 | Daisy | F | Eye of the day | Old English | 1786 |
| 383 | Peter | M | Rock | Latin | 1777 |
| 384 | Charlie | M | Manly | English | 1776 |
| 385 | Kyrie | M | | | 1774 |
| 386 | Thiago | M | | | 1765 |
| 387 | Brian | M | Honorable | Irish | 1763 |
| 388 | Kenneth | M | Handsome | Irish | 1751 |
| 389 | Andres | M | Manly | Greek | 1750 |

| 390 | Reese | F | Ardor | Welsh | 1748 |
|---|---|---|---|---|---|
| 391 | Laila | F | Nightfall | Hebrew | 1735 |
| 392 | Mya | F | Emerald | Burmese | 1728 |
| 393 | Amy | F | Beloved | Latin | 1724 |
| 394 | Lukas | M | Bringer of light | Latin | 1723 |
| 395 | Teagan | F | Beautiful | Welsh | 1723 |
| 396 | Aidan | M | Little fiery one | Irish | 1718 |
| 397 | Amaya | F | | | 1709 |
| 398 | Jax | M | God has been gracious | American | 1707 |
| 399 | Elise | F | God is my oath | French | 1702 |
| 400 | Caden | M | Barrel | English | 1700 |
| 401 | Harmony | F | A state of order or agreement | Latin | 1694 |
| 402 | Paige | F | Attendant | French | 1690 |
| 403 | Milo | M | Merciful | German | 1688 |
| 404 | Paul | M | Small | Latin | 1684 |
| 405 | Beckett | M | | | 1678 |
| 406 | Brady | M | Dweller on the broad Island | Old English | 1676 |
| 407 | Adaline | F | Noble | French | 1673 |
| 408 | Fiona | F | Fair | Irish | 1672 |
| 409 | Colin | M | Victory of the people | Greek | 1662 |
| 410 | Alaina | F | Attractive | Irish | 1660 |
| 411 | Nicole | F | Victory of the people | French | 1654 |
| 412 | Genevieve | F | White wave | French | 1653 |
| 413 | Lucia | F | Bringer of light | Italian | 1651 |
| 414 | Alina | F | Beautiful | Scottish | 1650 |
| 415 | Mckenzie | F | Fair one | Irish | 1645 |
| 416 | Callie | F | Fortress | Greek | 1639 |
| 417 | Omar | M | Long Living | Arabic | 1639 |
| 418 | Bradley | M | Dweller at the broad meadow | Old English | 1638 |
| 419 | Javier | M | Owner of a new house | Spanish | 1638 |
| 420 | Payton | F | Noble woman | Irish | 1635 |
| 421 | Knox | M | From the hills | English | 1628 |
| 422 | Jaden | M | Stone of the side | English | 1627 |
| 423 | Eloise | F | Famous in war | French | 1621 |
| 424 | Brooke | F | A small stream | Old English | 1609 |
| 425 | Londyn | F | | | 1606 |

| 426 | Mariah | F | Bitter or sea of bitterness | Hebrew | 1604 |
|---|---|---|---|---|---|
| 427 | Barrett | M | Brave as a bear | German | 1601 |
| 428 | Julianna | F | | | 1593 |
| 429 | Rachel | F | Innocence of a lamb | Hebrew | 1591 |
| 430 | Daniela | F | God is my judge | Spanish | 1587 |
| 431 | Gracie | F | Beauty of form | Latin | 1586 |
| 432 | Israel | M | Contender with God | Hebrew | 1576 |
| 433 | Catherine | F | Pure | Greek | 1573 |
| 434 | Matias | M | Gift of God | Spanish | 1558 |
| 435 | Angelina | F | Messenger of God | English | 1550 |
| 436 | Jorge | M | Farmer | Greek | 1547 |
| 437 | Zander | M | Defender of mankind | Greek | 1546 |
| 438 | Derek | M | Ruler of the people | German | 1540 |
| 439 | Josue | M | God is salvation | French | 1532 |
| 440 | Presley | F | From the priest's meadow | Old English | 1526 |
| 441 | Cayden | M | | | 1525 |
| 442 | Josie | F | God will add | English | 1524 |
| 443 | Holden | M | From the hollow valley | Old English | 1518 |
| 444 | Harley | F | From the hare's meadow | English | 1515 |
| 445 | Adelyn | F | | | 1511 |
| 446 | Griffin | M | Hooked nose | Latin | 1511 |
| 447 | Vanessa | F | Butterfly | Greek | 1508 |
| 448 | Arthur | M | Noble | Irish | 1503 |
| 449 | Leon | M | Brave as a lion | German | 1503 |
| 450 | Felix | M | Fortunate or happy | Latin | 1498 |
| 451 | Remington | M | From the raven farm | English | 1497 |
| 452 | Makayla | F | Who is like God | Hebrew | 1492 |
| 453 | Jake | M | Supplanted | Hebrew | 1491 |
| 454 | Killian | M | Little Kelly | Irish | 1491 |
| 455 | Parker | F | Gamekeeper | English | 1487 |
| 456 | Juliette | F | Downy bearded or youthful | French | 1485 |
| 457 | Clayton | M | Settlement by the clay pit | Old English | 1482 |
| 458 | Amara | F | Eternally beautiful | Greek | 1478 |
| 459 | Sean | M | God is gracious | Irish | 1469 |

| 460 | Marley | F | From the lake meadow | English | 1463 |
|---|---|---|---|---|---|
| 461 | Adriel | M | From God's congregation | Hebrew | 1458 |
| 462 | Lila | F | Night | Arabic | 1456 |
| 463 | Riley | M | Dweller by the rye field | Old English | 1454 |
| 464 | Archer | M | Bowman | English | 1450 |
| 465 | Legend | M | | | 1448 |
| 466 | Ana | F | Grace | Spanish | 1443 |
| 467 | Rowan | F | From the rowan tree | English | 1440 |
| 468 | Alana | F | Attractive | Irish | 1432 |
| 469 | Erick | M | | | 1428 |
| 470 | Michelle | F | Who is like God | French | 1421 |
| 471 | Enzo | M | Ruler of the estate | German | 1419 |
| 472 | Malia | F | Bitter or sea of bitterness | Spanish | 1416 |
| 473 | Rebecca | F | Bound | Hebrew | 1416 |
| 474 | Corbin | M | Raven | Latin | 1412 |
| 475 | Brooklynn | F | Stream by the lake | English | 1410 |
| 476 | Brynlee | F | | | 1408 |
| 477 | Summer | F | The warmest season of the year | Old English | 1401 |
| 478 | Francisco | M | Free or from France | Spanish | 1398 |
| 479 | Sloane | F | Warrior | Irish | 1397 |
| 480 | Leila | F | Dark beauty | Hebrew | 1395 |
| 481 | Sienna | F | Reddish brown | Italian | 1392 |
| 482 | Dallas | M | Waterfall near the field | Scottish | 1389 |
| 483 | Adriana | F | Dark | Italian | 1387 |
| 484 | Sawyer | F | Wood cutter | English | 1385 |
| 485 | Kendall | F | Valley of the river Kent | Old English | 1384 |
| 486 | Emilio | M | Industrious | Italian/Spanish | 1383 |
| 487 | Gunner | M | Battle warrior | Scandinavian | 1383 |
| 488 | Juliet | F | Downy bearded or youthful | French | 1378 |
| 489 | Destiny | F | Fate | French | 1374 |
| 490 | Alayna | F | Attractive | Irish | 1373 |
| 491 | Elliana | F | | | 1370 |
| 492 | Simon | M | God is heard | Hebrew | 1366 |
| 493 | Diana | F | Divine | Latin | 1358 |

| | | | | | |
|---|---|---|---|---|---|
| 494 | Andre | M | Manly | French | 1356 |
| 495 | Walter | M | Army ruler | German | 1353 |
| 496 | Hayden | F | From the hedged valley | English | 1351 |
| 497 | Ayla | F | Oak tree | Hebrew | 1346 |
| 498 | Dakota | F | Allies or friends | Sioux | 1346 |
| 499 | Angela | F | Messenger | Latin | 1344 |
| 500 | Damien | M | To tame | Greek | 1340 |
| 501 | Noelle | F | Christmas | French | 1339 |
| 502 | Rosalie | F | | | 1339 |
| 503 | Joanna | F | God is gracious | English | 1337 |
| 504 | Jayla | F | Happy | Latin | 1334 |
| 505 | Chance | M | Church official | Old English | 1332 |
| 506 | Phoenix | M | Bright or red | Greek | 1332 |
| 507 | Alivia | F | | | 1330 |
| 508 | Colt | M | Young horse or frisky | English | 1329 |
| 509 | Lola | F | Sorrow of the Virgin Mary | Spanish | 1323 |
| 510 | Emersyn | F | | | 1322 |
| 511 | Tanner | M | Leather tanner | English | 1322 |
| 512 | Stephen | M | To wear a crown | Greek | 1321 |
| 513 | Kameron | M | Crooked nose | Scottish | 1320 |
| 514 | Tobias | M | The Lord is good | Hebrew | 1320 |
| 515 | Manuel | M | God is with us | Hebrew | 1319 |
| 516 | Amari | M | Immortal | Latin | 1313 |
| 517 | Emerson | M | Industrious ruler | German | 1310 |
| 518 | Georgia | F | Farmer | Greek | 1305 |
| 519 | Selena | F | Moon | Greek | 1296 |
| 520 | Louis | M | Famous warrior | German | 1290 |
| 521 | June | F | Sixth month of the year | Latin | 1288 |
| 522 | Daleyza | F | | | 1285 |
| 523 | Cody | M | Cushion | Old English | 1284 |
| 524 | Finley | M | | | 1284 |
| 525 | Tessa | F | Harvester | Greek | 1283 |
| 526 | Iker | M | Visitation | Basque | 1280 |
| 527 | Maggie | F | A pearl | Greek | 1278 |
| 528 | Martin | M | Warlike | Latin | 1276 |
| 529 | Rafael | M | God has healed | Hebrew | 1276 |
| 530 | Nash | M | | | 1273 |

| 531 | Jessica | F | He sees | Hebrew | 1271 |
|---|---|---|---|---|---|
| 532 | Beckham | M | | | 1263 |
| 533 | Remi | F | From the raven farm | English | 1262 |
| 534 | Cash | M | | | 1260 |
| 535 | Delaney | F | Son of the challenger | Irish | 1259 |
| 536 | Camille | F | Young ceremonial attendant | French | 1256 |
| 537 | Karson | M | | | 1256 |
| 538 | Vivienne | F | Full of life, lively or alive | French | 1255 |
| 539 | Rylan | M | Island meadow | Irish | 1253 |
| 540 | Hope | F | Expectation | Old English | 1250 |
| 541 | Mckenna | F | | | 1247 |
| 542 | Reid | M | Red hair or a ruddy complexion | Scottish | 1244 |
| 543 | Gemma | F | Precious stone | Latin | 1241 |
| 544 | Olive | F | Olive tree | Latin | 1241 |
| 545 | Alexandria | F | Defender of mankind | Greek | 1238 |
| 546 | Blakely | F | From the dark meadow | Old English | 1226 |
| 547 | Theo | M | | | 1223 |
| 548 | Ace | M | Unity | Latin | 1222 |
| 549 | Eduardo | M | Wealthy guardian | Spanish | 1221 |
| 550 | Izabella | F | Consecrated to God | Italian | 1220 |
| 551 | Catalina | F | Pure | Spanish | 1218 |
| 552 | Raegan | F | | | 1213 |
| 553 | Journee | F | | | 1212 |
| 554 | Gabrielle | F | God is my strength | French | 1210 |
| 555 | Spencer | M | Dispenser of provisions | Old English | 1200 |
| 556 | Lucille | F | Bringer of light | French | 1197 |
| 557 | Ruth | F | Companion | Hebrew | 1194 |
| 558 | Raymond | M | Wise protector | English | 1192 |
| 559 | Maximiliano | M | | | 1191 |
| 560 | Anderson | M | | | 1190 |
| 561 | Ronan | M | Little seal | Irish | 1190 |
| 562 | Amiyah | F | | | 1189 |
| 563 | Evangeline | F | Bringer of good news | Greek | 1186 |
| 564 | Blake | F | Dark complexioned | Old English | 1182 |
| 565 | Thea | F | Goddess | Greek | 1180 |
| 566 | Lane | M | A narrow country road | Old English | 1176 |

| 567 | Cristian | M | Follower of Christ or anointed | Greek | 1175 |
|-----|----------|---|-------------------------------|-------|------|
| 568 | Amina | F | Trustworthy | Arabic | 1170 |
| 569 | Giselle | F | Pledge | German | 1170 |
| 570 | Lilah | F | Night | Arabic | 1168 |
| 571 | Melissa | F | A bee | English | 1168 |
| 572 | River | F | Flowing water | French | 1166 |
| 573 | Titus | M | To honor | Latin | 1166 |
| 574 | Kate | F | Pure | Greek | 1162 |
| 575 | Travis | M | To cross the river | French | 1161 |
| 576 | Jett | M | A deep or glossy black | Greek | 1160 |
| 577 | Ricardo | M | Rich and powerful ruler | Spanish | 1160 |
| 578 | Adelaide | F | Noble | German | 1155 |
| 579 | Charlee | F | Strong and womanly | English | 1154 |
| 580 | Bodhi | M | | | 1154 |
| 581 | Vera | F | Faith or truth | Slavic | 1153 |
| 582 | Leia | F | Tired or weary | Hebrew | 1151 |
| 583 | Gabriela | F | God is my strength | Italian | 1149 |
| 584 | Zara | F | Princess | Hebrew | 1149 |
| 585 | Jane | F | God is gracious | English | 1148 |
| 586 | Journey | F | To travel | French | 1148 |
| 587 | Gideon | M | Tree cutter | Hebrew | 1145 |
| 588 | Elaina | F | Light | French | 1137 |
| 589 | Jaiden | M | Jade | Spanish | 1135 |
| 590 | Fernando | M | Adventurous and risky | Spanish | 1134 |
| 591 | Miriam | F | Sea of bitterness | Hebrew | 1134 |
| 592 | Briella | F | | | 1129 |
| 593 | Mario | M | Of the sea or sailor | Italian | 1129 |
| 594 | Conor | M | Exalted | Irish | 1127 |
| 595 | Stephanie | F | A crown of garland | French | 1126 |
| 596 | Cali | F | | | 1122 |
| 597 | Keegan | M | Little fire | Irish | 1113 |
| 598 | Ali | M | To ascend | Arabic | 1111 |
| 599 | Ember | F | To burn | Latin | 1111 |
| 600 | Lilliana | F | | | 1108 |
| 601 | Aniyah | F | | | 1107 |
| 602 | Logan | F | Dweller in a little hollow | Irish | 1103 |
| 603 | Kamila | F | Perfection | Arabic | 1100 |

| 604 | Cesar | M | Hairy | Latin | 1099 |
|---|---|---|---|---|---|
| 605 | Ellis | M | The Lord is my God | English | 1099 |
| 606 | Jayceon | M | | | 1097 |
| 607 | Walker | M | To roll | Old English | 1096 |
| 608 | Cohen | M | | | 1094 |
| 609 | Brynn | F | | | 1091 |
| 610 | Ariella | F | | | 1090 |
| 611 | Makenzie | F | | | 1088 |
| 612 | Annie | F | Gracious | English | 1087 |
| 613 | Arlo | M | Fortified hill | English | 1084 |
| 614 | Mariana | F | Bitter or sea of bitterness | Spanish | 1084 |
| 615 | Kali | F | Flower bud | Greek | 1083 |
| 616 | Haven | F | A refuge or shelter | Old English | 1080 |
| 617 | Elsie | F | God is my oath | Hebrew | 1077 |
| 618 | Nyla | F | | | 1076 |
| 619 | Paris | F | Lover | Greek | 1076 |
| 620 | Lena | F | Sun ray | Greek | 1072 |
| 621 | Hector | M | Steadfast | Greek | 1070 |
| 622 | Dante | M | Enduring | Latin | 1069 |
| 623 | Freya | F | Goddess of fertility | Norse | 1069 |
| 624 | Kyler | M | Land where cattle graze | Scottish | 1064 |
| 625 | Adelynn | F | Noble | English | 1063 |
| 626 | Lyric | F | Expression of emotion | Greek | 1057 |
| 627 | Garrett | M | Mighty with a spear | Irish | 1056 |
| 628 | Donovan | M | Dark warrior | Irish | 1051 |
| 629 | Seth | M | Appointed | Hebrew | 1051 |
| 630 | Jeffrey | M | Divinely peaceful | Old English | 1049 |
| 631 | Camilla | F | Young ceremonial attendant | Italian | 1047 |
| 632 | Tyson | M | Firebrand | French | 1045 |
| 633 | Sage | F | Wise | Latin | 1043 |
| 634 | Jase | M | | | 1042 |
| 635 | Jennifer | F | White wave | Welsh | 1042 |
| 636 | Paislee | F | | | 1041 |
| 637 | Talia | F | Lamb | Hebrew | 1040 |
| 638 | Desmond | M | From south Munster | Irish | 1039 |
| 639 | Caiden | M | | | 1038 |

| 640 | Gage | M | Measure | French | 1035 |
|---|---|---|---|---|---|
| 641 | Alessandra | F | Defender of mankind | Italian | 1034 |
| 642 | Atlas | M | | | 1034 |
| 643 | Major | M | | | 1034 |
| 644 | Juniper | F | | | 1033 |
| 645 | Fatima | F | To abstain | Arabic | 1031 |
| 646 | Devin | M | Poet | Irish | 1030 |
| 647 | Edwin | M | Prosperous friend | Old English | 1027 |
| 648 | Angelo | M | Messenger | Latin | 1020 |
| 649 | Raelyn | F | | | 1019 |
| 650 | Orion | M | Son of fire | Greek | 1015 |
| 651 | Amira | F | Speech | Hebrew | 1014 |
| 652 | Arielle | F | Lion of God | Hebrew | 1013 |
| 653 | Phoebe | F | Bright one | Greek | 1012 |
| 654 | Kinley | F | | | 1010 |
| 655 | Ada | F | Wealthy | English | 1009 |
| 656 | Nina | F | Full of grace | Russian | 1009 |
| 657 | Ariah | F | | | 1005 |
| 658 | Conner | M | Exalted | Irish | 1005 |
| 659 | Samara | F | Protected by God | Latin | 1002 |
| 660 | Julius | M | Downy bearded or youthful | Latin | 1001 |
| 661 | Marco | M | Warlike | Italian | 1001 |
| 662 | Jensen | M | | | 999 |
| 663 | Myla | F | Merciful | English | 997 |
| 664 | Brinley | F | | | 996 |
| 665 | Cassidy | F | Clever or curly headed | Irish | 995 |
| 666 | Maci | F | Weapon | French | 995 |
| 667 | Daxton | M | French town Dax | French | 992 |
| 668 | Peyton | M | Warrior's town | Old English | 992 |
| 669 | Aspen | F | A tree | English | 990 |
| 670 | Zayn | M | | | 988 |
| 671 | Allie | F | | | 987 |
| 672 | Collin | M | Victory of the people | Greek | 987 |
| 673 | Jaylen | M | | | 985 |
| 674 | Dakota | M | Allies or friends | Sioux | 984 |
| 675 | Keira | F | Little dark haired one | Irish | 984 |
| 676 | Kaia | F | | | 978 |

| 677 | Prince | M | Prince | Latin | 978 |
|---|---|---|---|---|---|
| 678 | Makenna | F | | | 971 |
| 679 | Johnny | M | God is gracious | Hebrew | 964 |
| 680 | Kayson | M | | | 964 |
| 681 | Cruz | M | Cross | Spanish | 961 |
| 682 | Hendrix | M | | | 960 |
| 683 | Amanda | F | Lovable, worthy to be loved | Latin | 954 |
| 684 | Heaven | F | Paradise | English | 954 |
| 685 | Joy | F | Rejoicing | Latin | 954 |
| 686 | Atticus | M | | | 953 |
| 687 | Troy | M | Foot soldier | Irish | 949 |
| 688 | Lia | F | Bringer of good news | Greek | 948 |
| 689 | Madilyn | F | | | 946 |
| 690 | Gracelyn | F | | | 942 |
| 691 | Kane | M | Tribute | Irish | 940 |
| 692 | Laura | F | Crowned with laurels | Latin | 939 |
| 693 | Edgar | M | Lucky spearman | Old English | 938 |
| 694 | Evelynn | F | Hazelnut | Old English | 938 |
| 695 | Lexi | F | Defender of mankind | Greek | 938 |
| 696 | Haley | F | Heroine | Scandinavian | 937 |
| 697 | Sergio | M | Attendant | Italian | 937 |
| 698 | Kash | M | | | 934 |
| 699 | Miranda | F | To be admired | Latin | 934 |
| 700 | Marshall | M | Steward | French | 932 |
| 701 | Johnathan | M | Gift of God | Hebrew | 929 |
| 702 | Kaitlyn | F | Pure | Irish | 929 |
| 703 | Daniella | F | | | 927 |
| 704 | Felicity | F | Fortunate or happy | English | 926 |
| 705 | Jacqueline | F | Supplanted | French | 920 |
| 706 | Evie | F | Living one | Hebrew | 919 |
| 707 | Angel | F | Messenger | Latin | 917 |
| 708 | Romeo | M | Pilgrim to Rome | Italian | 913 |
| 709 | Shane | M | God is gracious | Irish | 909 |
| 710 | Warren | M | A game preserve | French | 907 |
| 711 | Danielle | F | God is my judge | Hebrew | 906 |
| 712 | Joaquin | M | God shall establish | Spanish | 901 |

| 713 | Wade | M | River ford | Old English | 899 |
|---|---|---|---|---|---|
| 714 | Ainsley | F | My own meadow | Scottish | 898 |
| 715 | Leonel | M | Young lion | English | 898 |
| 716 | Trevor | M | Prudent | Irish | 898 |
| 717 | Dominick | M | | | 897 |
| 718 | Muhammad | M | Praiseworthy | Arabic | 896 |
| 719 | Erik | M | Eternal ruler | Old Norse | 895 |
| 720 | Odin | M | God of all | Old Norse | 893 |
| 721 | Quinn | M | Queen | Old English | 892 |
| 722 | Dylan | F | Son of the sea | Welsh | 890 |
| 723 | Jaxton | M | | | 888 |
| 724 | Dalton | M | Town in the valley | Old English | 886 |
| 725 | Kiara | F | Dark | Irish | 885 |
| 726 | Millie | F | Industrious | English | 885 |
| 727 | Jordan | F | To flow down or descend | Hebrew | 882 |
| 728 | Nehemiah | M | Comforted by God | Hebrew | 882 |
| 729 | Frank | M | Free or from France | English | 881 |
| 730 | Grady | M | Noble | Irish | 881 |
| 731 | Gregory | M | Vigilant watchman | Latin | 881 |
| 732 | Andy | M | Manly | Greek | 875 |
| 733 | Maddison | F | | | 875 |
| 734 | Rylie | F | | | 875 |
| 735 | Solomon | M | Peaceful | Hebrew | 868 |
| 736 | Malik | M | Master or sovereign | Arabic | 862 |
| 737 | Alicia | F | Truthful | English | 861 |
| 738 | Maeve | F | Joy | Irish | 860 |
| 739 | Rory | M | Red ruler | Irish | 856 |
| 740 | Clark | M | Clergyman or cleric | Old English | 855 |
| 741 | Margot | F | Pearl | French | 854 |
| 742 | Kylee | F | Beautiful | Irish | 853 |
| 743 | Phoenix | F | Bright or red | Greek | 852 |
| 744 | Reed | M | Redheaded | English | 852 |
| 745 | Harvey | M | Army warrior | German | 850 |
| 746 | Heidi | F | Noble and serene | German | 850 |
| 747 | Zuri | F | White or light skinned | Basque | 847 |
| 748 | Zayne | M | God is Gracious | English | 846 |
| 749 | Jay | M | Blue jay | French | 845 |

| 750 | Alondra | F | Defender of mankind | Greek | 844 |
|---|---|---|---|---|---|
| 751 | Lana | F | Attractive | Irish | 842 |
| 752 | Madeleine | F | From the high tower | French | 841 |
| 753 | Jared | M | Descending | Hebrew | 839 |
| 754 | Gracelynn | F | | | 835 |
| 755 | Kenzie | F | The fair one | Scottish | 835 |
| 756 | Miracle | F | An amazing wonder | Latin | 831 |
| 757 | Noel | M | Christmas | French | 831 |
| 758 | Shelby | F | The place where willows grow | English | 831 |
| 759 | Elle | F | Feminine | French | 828 |
| 760 | Adrianna | F | Dark | Italian | 827 |
| 761 | Bianca | F | White | Italian | 827 |
| 762 | Addilyn | F | | | 821 |
| 763 | Shawn | M | God is gracious | Irish | 821 |
| 764 | Fabian | M | Bean grower | Latin | 819 |
| 765 | Kira | F | Lord or master | Greek | 817 |
| 766 | Veronica | F | One who brings victory or true image | Latin | 817 |
| 767 | Gwendolyn | F | White wave | Welsh | 816 |
| 768 | Esmeralda | F | Emerald | Spanish | 815 |
| 769 | Ibrahim | M | My father is exalted | Arabic | 814 |
| 770 | Chelsea | F | Port or landing place | Old English | 813 |
| 771 | Alison | F | Truthful | Old English | 812 |
| 772 | Skyler | F | The isle of Skye | Scottish | 812 |
| 773 | Adonis | M | Handsome | Greek | 809 |
| 774 | Ismael | M | God listens | Arabic | 809 |
| 775 | Pedro | M | Rock | Spanish | 809 |
| 776 | Leland | M | From the meadow land | Old English | 808 |
| 777 | Magnolia | F | Flowering tree | Latin | 808 |
| 778 | Daphne | F | Laurel | Greek | 807 |
| 779 | Jenna | F | Paradise | Arabic | 804 |
| 780 | Malakai | M | | | 804 |
| 781 | Malcolm | M | Servant | Scottish | 804 |
| 782 | Alexis | M | Defender of mankind | Greek | 803 |
| 783 | Everleigh | F | From Ever's meadow | English | 803 |
| 784 | Kason | M | | | 802 |
| 785 | Kyla | F | Victorious | Unknown | 802 |

| 786 | Porter | M | Gatekeeper | Latin | 799 |
|---|---|---|---|---|---|
| 787 | Braelynn | F | | | 795 |
| 788 | Harlow | F | From the hare's hill | English | 794 |
| 789 | Annalise | F | Full of grace | German | 792 |
| 790 | Mikayla | F | Who is like God | Hebrew | 792 |
| 791 | Sullivan | M | Dark eyes | Irish | 792 |
| 792 | Dahlia | F | | | 790 |
| 793 | Raiden | M | | | 789 |
| 794 | Allen | M | Handsome | Irish | 787 |
| 795 | Maliyah | F | | | 786 |
| 796 | Ari | M | Lion | Hebrew | 785 |
| 797 | Averie | F | | | 784 |
| 798 | Scarlet | F | Bright red | English | 783 |
| 799 | Kayleigh | F | Pure | American | 782 |
| 800 | Luciana | F | | | 782 |
| 801 | Russell | M | Red haired | French | 782 |
| 802 | Princeton | M | Prince's town | Old English | 781 |
| 803 | Kelsey | F | Ship island | Scottish | 780 |
| 804 | Nadia | F | Hope | Russian | 777 |
| 805 | Winston | M | From the friendly town | Old English | 777 |
| 806 | Amber | F | A jewel | Arabic | 776 |
| 807 | Gia | F | God is gracious | Italian | 776 |
| 808 | Kamryn | F | Crooked nose | American | 774 |
| 809 | Yaretzi | F | | | 773 |
| 810 | Carmen | F | Song | Latin | 772 |
| 811 | Jimena | F | Heard | Spanish | 772 |
| 812 | Kendrick | M | Royal ruler | Scottish | 772 |
| 813 | Erin | F | Ireland | Irish | 771 |
| 814 | Roberto | M | Bright with fame | Spanish | 771 |
| 815 | Christina | F | Follower of Christ or anointed | Greek | 770 |
| 816 | Katie | F | Pure | English | 770 |
| 817 | Ryan | F | Little king | Irish | 770 |
| 818 | Viviana | F | Full of life, lively or alive | French | 769 |
| 819 | Alexia | F | Defender of mankind | Greek | 768 |
| 820 | Anaya | F | | | 764 |
| 821 | Lennox | M | With many elm trees | Scottish | 762 |
| 822 | Serena | F | Calm or peaceful | Latin | 761 |

| 823 | Hayes | M | From the hedged land | English | 760 |
|---|---|---|---|---|---|
| 824 | Katelyn | F | Pure | Irish | 760 |
| 825 | Ophelia | F | Helper | Greek | 760 |
| 826 | Regina | F | Queen | Latin | 759 |
| 827 | Finnegan | M | Light skinned | Irish | 758 |
| 828 | Helen | F | Light | Greek | 758 |
| 829 | Remington | F | From the raven farm | English | 754 |
| 830 | Camryn | F | | | 752 |
| 831 | Nasir | M | | | 749 |
| 832 | Kade | M | Barrel | Old English | 748 |
| 833 | Cadence | F | Rhythm | Latin | 747 |
| 834 | Nico | M | Victory of the people | Greek | 747 |
| 835 | Royalty | F | | | 747 |
| 836 | Emanuel | M | God is with us | Hebrew | 746 |
| 837 | Landen | M | | | 746 |
| 838 | Amari | F | Immortal | Latin | 745 |
| 839 | Moises | M | Saved from the water | Hebrew | 745 |
| 840 | Ruben | M | Behold or a son | Hebrew | 745 |
| 841 | Hugo | M | Bright mind | Latin | 744 |
| 842 | Kathryn | F | Pure | English | 744 |
| 843 | Skye | F | The isle of Skye | Scottish | 744 |
| 844 | Jada | F | Stone of the side | Spanish | 743 |
| 845 | Emely | F | | | 743 |
| 846 | Ariyah | F | | | 740 |
| 847 | Abram | M | Exalted father | Hebrew | 739 |
| 848 | Adan | M | Of the red earth | Unknown | 739 |
| 849 | Aylin | F | | | 737 |
| 850 | Saylor | F | | | 735 |
| 851 | Kendra | F | Knowing | Old English | 734 |
| 852 | Cheyenne | F | Tribal name | American | 733 |
| 853 | Fernanda | F | Adventurous | German | 732 |
| 854 | Sabrina | F | From the border | Latin | 732 |
| 855 | Francesca | F | Free or from France | Italian | 730 |
| 856 | Khalil | M | Best friend | Arabic | 729 |
| 857 | Zaiden | M | | | 729 |
| 858 | Augustus | M | Majestic | Latin | 728 |
| 859 | Eve | F | Life | Hebrew | 727 |

| 860 | Marcos | M | Warlike | Spanish | 725 |
|---|---|---|---|---|---|
| 861 | Philip | M | Lover of horses | Latin | 725 |
| 862 | Phillip | M | Lover of horses | Greek | 725 |
| 863 | Cyrus | M | Lord | Greek | 724 |
| 864 | Esteban | M | Crowned | Spanish | 724 |
| 865 | Mckinley | F | | | 724 |
| 866 | Frances | F | Free or from France | Latin | 723 |
| 867 | Braylen | M | | | 717 |
| 868 | Sarai | F | Argumentative | Hebrew | 717 |
| 869 | Carolina | F | Little and womanly | Italian | 715 |
| 870 | Albert | M | Noble and bright | German | 714 |
| 871 | Bruce | M | Woods | French | 714 |
| 872 | Kamden | M | From the winding Valley | Celtic | 714 |
| 873 | Kennedi | F | | | 713 |
| 874 | Nylah | F | | | 711 |
| 875 | Tatum | F | Light hearted | English | 710 |
| 876 | Lawson | M | Son of Law or Lawrence | English | 708 |
| 877 | Alani | F | Attractive | Irish | 705 |
| 878 | Jamison | M | Supplanted | English | 705 |
| 879 | Lennon | F | Small cloak or cape | Irish | 705 |
| 880 | Sterling | M | Of high quality or pure | Old English | 705 |
| 881 | Damon | M | To tame | Greek | 704 |
| 882 | Gunnar | M | Battle warrior | Old Norse | 703 |
| 883 | Raven | F | Blackbird | Old English | 703 |
| 884 | Zariah | F | | | 703 |
| 885 | Kyson | M | | | 702 |
| 886 | Luka | M | | | 702 |
| 887 | Leslie | F | From the gray fortress | Scottish | 701 |
| 888 | Franklin | M | Free landowner | English | 700 |
| 889 | Ezequiel | M | Strength of God | Spanish | 699 |
| 890 | Winter | F | Born in the winter | Old English | 699 |
| 891 | Abby | F | My father rejoices | Hebrew | 696 |
| 892 | Mabel | F | | | 696 |
| 893 | Pablo | M | Small | Spanish | 696 |
| 894 | Sierra | F | Mountain | Spanish | 696 |
| 895 | Derrick | M | Ruler of the people | German | 694 |
| 896 | Zachariah | M | God remembers | Hebrew | 694 |

| 897 | Cade | M | Barrel | English | 693 |
|---|---|---|---|---|---|
| 898 | April | F | Second | Latin | 691 |
| 899 | Willa | F | Resolute protector | German | 691 |
| 900 | Carly | F | | | 687 |
| 901 | Jolene | F | God will add | Hebrew | 687 |
| 902 | Jonas | M | Dove | Hebrew | 687 |
| 903 | Rosemary | F | Bitter rose | English | 687 |
| 904 | Aviana | F | Bearer of good news | Greek | 686 |
| 905 | Madelynn | F | From the high tower | Greek | 685 |
| 906 | Selah | F | | | 684 |
| 907 | Renata | F | Reborn | Italian | 682 |
| 908 | Dexter | M | | | 681 |
| 909 | Lorelei | F | Alluring | German | 680 |
| 910 | Kolton | M | Coal town | English | 679 |
| 911 | Remy | M | From the raven farm | English | 678 |
| 912 | Hank | M | Ruler of the estate | American | 677 |
| 913 | Tate | M | Light hearted | Old English | 677 |
| 914 | Briana | F | Strong | Irish | 676 |
| 915 | Trenton | M | Trent's town | Old English | 673 |
| 916 | Celeste | F | Heavenly | Latin | 671 |
| 917 | Kian | M | Archaic | Unknown | 670 |
| 918 | Drew | M | Manly | English | 669 |
| 919 | Wren | F | | | 668 |
| 920 | Charleigh | F | | | 667 |
| 921 | Leighton | F | From the meadow farm | Old English | 665 |
| 922 | Annabella | F | Beautiful grace | Old English | 663 |
| 923 | Jayleen | F | | | 662 |
| 924 | Mohamed | M | Praiseworthy | Arabic | 662 |
| 925 | Dax | M | Water | French | 661 |
| 926 | Braelyn | F | | | 661 |
| 927 | Rocco | M | | | 661 |
| 928 | Ashlyn | F | Ash tree pool | English | 659 |
| 929 | Jazlyn | F | Fragrant flower | American | 659 |
| 930 | Mira | F | Admirable | Latin | 659 |
| 931 | Bowen | M | Son of Owen | Welsh | 658 |
| 932 | Mathias | M | Gift of God | Greek | 657 |
| 933 | Ronald | M | Rules with good judgment | Scottish | 655 |

| 934 | Oakley | F | From the oak tree meadow | English | 653 |
|---|---|---|---|---|---|
| 935 | Malaysia | F | | | 652 |
| 936 | Francis | M | Free or from France | Latin | 651 |
| 937 | Edith | F | Prosperous in war | Old English | 649 |
| 938 | Matthias | M | Gift from God | Hebrew | 649 |
| 939 | Milan | M | | | 649 |
| 940 | Maximilian | M | The greatest | Latin | 647 |
| 941 | Royce | M | Kingly | French | 647 |
| 942 | Skyler | M | The isle of Skye | Scottish | 647 |
| 943 | Avianna | F | Bearer of good news | Greek | 646 |
| 944 | Maryam | F | | | 645 |
| 945 | Corey | M | Dweller near a hollow | Irish | 644 |
| 946 | Emmalyn | F | Industrious | American | 644 |
| 947 | Hattie | F | Ruler of an enclosure | English | 643 |
| 948 | Kensley | F | | | 643 |
| 949 | Kasen | M | Protected with a helmet | Basque | 640 |
| 950 | Macie | F | Weapon | French | 640 |
| 951 | Drake | M | Dragon | English | 638 |
| 952 | Bristol | F | | | 638 |
| 953 | Marlee | F | | | 638 |
| 954 | Demi | F | Half | French | 637 |
| 955 | Cataleya | F | | | 636 |
| 956 | Maia | F | Close to God | Hebrew | 636 |
| 957 | Sylvia | F | Of the woods | Latin | 636 |
| 958 | Gerardo | M | Brave with a spear | Spanish | 635 |
| 959 | Itzel | F | | | 635 |
| 960 | Allyson | F | Truthful | Old English | 634 |
| 961 | Lilith | F | Of the night | Arabic | 633 |
| 962 | Melany | F | | | 632 |
| 963 | Jayson | M | | | 630 |
| 964 | Kaydence | F | | | 630 |
| 965 | Holly | F | To prick | Old English | 629 |
| 966 | Nayeli | F | | | 628 |
| 967 | Meredith | F | Protector of the sea | Welsh | 626 |
| 968 | Nia | F | Female champion | Irish | 626 |
| 969 | Sage | M | Wise | Latin | 626 |
| 970 | Liana | F | To bind or twine around | French | 625 |

| | Name | S | Meaning | Origin | Births |
|---|---|---|---|---|---|
| 971 | Megan | F | Pearl | Irish | 624 |
| 972 | Braylon | M | | | 621 |
| 973 | Justice | F | Just | Latin | 621 |
| 974 | Benson | M | Born of the right hand | Hebrew | 620 |
| 975 | Bethany | F | House of figs | Hebrew | 618 |
| 976 | Moses | M | Drawn out of the water | Hebrew | 618 |
| 977 | Alejandra | F | Defender of mankind | Spanish | 617 |
| 978 | Janelle | F | God is gracious | French | 617 |
| 979 | Alijah | M | | | 615 |
| 980 | Elisa | F | God is my oath | Greek | 615 |
| 981 | Adelina | F | Noble | English | 614 |
| 982 | Ashlynn | F | Ash tree pool | English | 614 |
| 983 | Elianna | F | | | 614 |
| 984 | Rhys | M | | | 614 |
| 985 | Aleah | F | | | 612 |
| 986 | Myra | F | Sweet ointment | Latin | 612 |
| 987 | Otto | M | Wealthy or prosperous | German | 612 |
| 988 | Lainey | F | | | 610 |
| 989 | Oakley | M | From the oak tree meadow | English | 610 |
| 990 | Blair | F | Dweller on the plain | Scottish | 609 |
| 991 | Kassidy | F | Clever | Irish | 609 |
| 992 | Charley | F | Manly | English | 608 |
| 993 | Virginia | F | Pure | Latin | 608 |
| 994 | Armando | M | Soldier | Spanish | 606 |
| 995 | Kara | F | Graceful or beautiful | Greek | 606 |
| 996 | Jaime | M | Supplanted | Hebrew | 604 |
| 997 | Nixon | M | Son of Nick | English | 603 |
| 998 | Saul | M | Asked of God | Hebrew | 603 |
| 999 | Scott | M | From Scotland | Old English | 602 |
| 1000 | Brycen | M | Son of the strong one | Welsh | 601 |

# TOP 1001 TO 2000 NAMES IN THE U.S.

| | Name | S | Meaning | Origin | Births |
|---|---|---|---|---|---|
| 1001 | Helena | F | Light | Greek | 600 |

| 1002 | Sasha | F | Defender of mankind | Russian | 600 |
|------|-------|---|---------------------|---------|-----|
| 1003 | Ariel | M | Lion of God | Hebrew | 599 |
| 1004 | Julie | F | Downy bearded or youthful | English | 599 |
| 1005 | Michaela | F | Who is like God | Hebrew | 599 |
| 1006 | Carter | F | Transporter of goods with a cart | Old English | 598 |
| 1007 | Enrique | M | Ruler of the estate | Spanish | 597 |
| 1008 | Matilda | F | Mighty battle maiden | German | 597 |
| 1009 | Kehlani | F | | | 596 |
| 1010 | Donald | M | World ruler | Scottish | 594 |
| 1011 | Henley | F | | | 594 |
| 1012 | Maisie | F | Pearl | Scottish | 594 |
| 1013 | Hallie | F | Heroine | Scandinavian | 592 |
| 1014 | Chandler | M | Maker of candles | Old English | 590 |
| 1015 | Asa | M | Healer | Hebrew | 588 |
| 1016 | Jazmin | F | | | 588 |
| 1017 | Priscilla | F | Ancient, old or primitive | Latin | 587 |
| 1018 | Eden | M | Delight | Hebrew | 586 |
| 1019 | Davis | M | Son of David | Welsh | 582 |
| 1020 | Keith | M | Of the forest | Scottish | 582 |
| 1021 | Frederick | M | Peaceful ruler | German | 580 |
| 1022 | Marilyn | F | Bitter or sea of bitterness | Hebrew | 580 |
| 1023 | Rowen | M | Red haired | English | 580 |
| 1024 | Danna | F | God is my judge | Hebrew | 579 |
| 1025 | Cecelia | F | | | 579 |
| 1026 | Lawrence | M | Crowned with laurels | Latin | 579 |
| 1027 | Leonidas | M | | | 579 |
| 1028 | Aden | M | | | 578 |
| 1029 | Colette | F | Victory of the people | French | 578 |
| 1030 | Julio | M | Downy bearded or youthful | Spanish | 578 |
| 1031 | Baylee | F | Law enforcer or bailiff | Old English | 577 |
| 1032 | Darius | M | Wealthy | Greek | 577 |
| 1033 | Johan | M | God is gracious | German | 576 |
| 1034 | Deacon | M | One who serves | Greek | 575 |
| 1035 | Elliott | F | Jehovah is God | French | 575 |
| 1036 | Ivanna | F | God is gracious | Slavic | 575 |
| 1037 | Cameron | F | Crooked nose | Scottish | 574 |

| 1038 | Celine | F | Blind | French | 574 |
|------|--------|---|-------|--------|-----|
| 1039 | Alayah | F | | | 573 |
| 1040 | Danny | M | God is my judge | Hebrew | 572 |
| 1041 | Hanna | F | Gracious | Hebrew | 572 |
| 1042 | Cason | M | | | 572 |
| 1043 | Imani | F | Believer or faith | Arabic | 572 |
| 1044 | Nikolai | M | Victory of the people | Russian | 571 |
| 1045 | Taylor | M | To cut | French | 571 |
| 1046 | Angelica | F | Like an angel | Greek | 570 |
| 1047 | Alec | M | Defender of mankind | Scottish | 569 |
| 1048 | Royal | M | Regal | French | 569 |
| 1049 | Armani | M | | | 567 |
| 1050 | Kieran | M | Little and dark | Irish | 566 |
| 1051 | Luciano | M | Bringer of light | Italian | 566 |
| 1052 | Emelia | F | | | 565 |
| 1053 | Kalani | F | The heavens | Hawaiian | 565 |
| 1054 | Omari | M | | | 565 |
| 1055 | Rodrigo | M | Famous ruler | Spanish | 564 |
| 1056 | Alanna | F | Attractive | Irish | 563 |
| 1057 | Lorelai | F | | | 563 |
| 1058 | Macy | F | Weapon | French | 563 |
| 1059 | Karina | F | Beloved | Latin | 562 |
| 1060 | Aleena | F | Fair | Celtic | 561 |
| 1061 | Addyson | F | | | 561 |
| 1062 | Arjun | M | | | 560 |
| 1063 | Aisha | F | Lively | Arabic | 559 |
| 1064 | Johanna | F | God is gracious | German | 559 |
| 1065 | Ahmed | M | Much praised | Arabic | 558 |
| 1066 | Mallory | F | Unfortunate or unlucky | French | 556 |
| 1067 | Brendan | M | Little raven | Irish | 555 |
| 1068 | Cullen | M | Handsome | Irish | 555 |
| 1069 | Leona | F | Brave as a lioness | German | 555 |
| 1070 | Raul | M | Wolf counselled | French | 555 |
| 1071 | Mariam | F | Bitter or sea of bitterness | Hebrew | 554 |
| 1072 | Raphael | M | God has healed | Hebrew | 554 |
| 1073 | Ronin | M | | | 554 |
| 1074 | Kynlee | F | | | 553 |

| 1075 | Madilynn | F |  |  | 553 |
|------|----------|---|--|--|-----|
| 1076 | Karen | F | Pure | Greek | 552 |
| 1077 | Karla | F | Farmer | German | 552 |
| 1078 | Brock | M | Badger | Old English | 547 |
| 1079 | Skyla | F |  |  | 547 |
| 1080 | Beatrice | F | She who brings happiness | Latin | 544 |
| 1081 | Pierce | M | Rock | French | 544 |
| 1082 | Alonzo | M | Eager for battle | Spanish | 543 |
| 1083 | Dayana | F |  |  | 543 |
| 1084 | Casey | M | Brave | Irish | 540 |
| 1085 | Dillon | M | Faithful or loyal | Irish | 540 |
| 1086 | Gloria | F | Glory | Latin | 538 |
| 1087 | Uriel | M | God is my light | Hebrew | 537 |
| 1088 | Milani | F |  |  | 536 |
| 1089 | Savanna | F | From the open plain | Spanish | 534 |
| 1090 | Dustin | M | Valiant fighter | German | 533 |
| 1091 | Karsyn | F | Marsh or mossy place | American | 533 |
| 1092 | Gianni | M | God is gracious | Italian | 532 |
| 1093 | Rory | F | Red ruler | Irish | 532 |
| 1094 | Roland | M | Famous in the land | German | 531 |
| 1095 | Giuliana | F |  |  | 530 |
| 1096 | Lauryn | F | Crowned with laurels | English | 530 |
| 1097 | Landyn | M |  |  | 528 |
| 1098 | Liberty | F | Free | Latin | 528 |
| 1099 | Galilea | F |  |  | 527 |
| 1100 | Kobe | M | Supplanted | Polish | 527 |
| 1101 | Aubrie | F | Blond ruler | French | 526 |
| 1102 | Charli | F | Strong and womanly | English | 526 |
| 1103 | Dorian | M | Mountainous region of Greece | English | 526 |
| 1104 | Emmitt | M |  |  | 526 |
| 1105 | Ryland | M | Island meadow | Irish | 526 |
| 1106 | Apollo | M | Manly | Greek | 525 |
| 1107 | Aarav | M |  |  | 524 |
| 1108 | Kyleigh | F |  |  | 524 |
| 1109 | Brylee | F |  |  | 523 |
| 1110 | Jillian | F | Youthful | Latin | 523 |

| 1111 | Anne | F | Gracious | Hebrew | 522 |
|---|---|---|---|---|---|
| 1112 | Roy | M | King | French | 522 |
| 1113 | Duke | M | Leader | French | 520 |
| 1114 | Haylee | F | | | 520 |
| 1115 | Dallas | F | Waterfall near the field | Scottish | 519 |
| 1116 | Azalea | F | Flower | Greek | 518 |
| 1117 | Jayda | F | | | 518 |
| 1118 | Quentin | M | The fifth | Latin | 518 |
| 1119 | Sam | M | Heard by God | Hebrew | 518 |
| 1120 | Tiffany | F | Epiphany | French | 516 |
| 1121 | Lewis | M | Famous or renowned fighter | English | 515 |
| 1122 | Avah | F | Like a bird | Latin | 514 |
| 1123 | Shiloh | F | God's Gift | Hebrew | 514 |
| 1124 | Tony | M | Flourishing | Greek | 514 |
| 1125 | Bailee | F | Law enforcer or bailiff | Old English | 513 |
| 1126 | Jazmine | F | Fragrant flower | Arabic | 511 |
| 1127 | Uriah | M | God is my light | Hebrew | 511 |
| 1128 | Dennis | M | God of wine | Greek | 510 |
| 1129 | Esme | F | Emerald | French | 510 |
| 1130 | Coraline | F | Maiden | English | 509 |
| 1131 | Madisyn | F | | | 508 |
| 1132 | Moshe | M | Drawn out of the water | Hebrew | 508 |
| 1133 | Elaine | F | Light | French | 506 |
| 1134 | Isaias | M | God is my salvation | Spanish | 506 |
| 1135 | Lilian | F | Lily | Latin | 506 |
| 1136 | Braden | M | Broad valley | Old English | 505 |
| 1137 | Kyra | F | Lord | Latin | 504 |
| 1138 | Kaliyah | F | | | 503 |
| 1139 | Kora | F | Maiden | Greek | 503 |
| 1140 | Octavia | F | Eighth | Italian | 502 |
| 1141 | Quinton | M | Fifth | Latin | 502 |
| 1142 | Cannon | M | | | 501 |
| 1143 | Irene | F | Peace | Greek | 501 |
| 1144 | Ayaan | M | | | 500 |
| 1145 | Kelly | F | Warrior | Irish | 500 |
| 1146 | Lacey | F | Cheerful | Latin | 500 |
| 1147 | Laurel | F | Laurel tree | Latin | 500 |

| 1148 | Adley | F | Judicious | Hebrew | 499 |
|------|-------|---|-----------|--------|-----|
| 1149 | Anika | F | Grace | Czech | 499 |
| 1150 | Janiyah | F | | | 499 |
| 1151 | Mathew | M | Gift of God | Hebrew | 499 |
| 1152 | Dorothy | F | Gift of God | Greek | 498 |
| 1153 | Kellan | M | | | 498 |
| 1154 | Niko | M | Victory of the people | Greek | 498 |
| 1155 | Sutton | F | From the south farm | English | 498 |
| 1156 | Julieta | F | Downy bearded or youthful | Spanish | 497 |
| 1157 | Kimber | F | | | 497 |
| 1158 | Remy | F | From the raven farm | English | 497 |
| 1159 | Cassandra | F | Doom | Greek | 496 |
| 1160 | Rebekah | F | Bound | Hebrew | 495 |
| 1161 | Collins | F | Victory of the people | Greek | 493 |
| 1162 | Edison | M | Son of Edward | English | 493 |
| 1163 | Elliot | F | Jehovah is God | French | 493 |
| 1164 | Emmy | F | Industrious | German | 493 |
| 1165 | Sloan | F | Warrior | Irish | 493 |
| 1166 | Hayley | F | From the hay meadow | English | 492 |
| 1167 | Amalia | F | Industrious | German | 491 |
| 1168 | Jemma | F | Little dove | Hebrew | 491 |
| 1169 | Izaiah | M | | | 489 |
| 1170 | Jamie | F | Supplanted | English | 488 |
| 1171 | Jerry | M | Mighty spearman | German | 488 |
| 1172 | Melina | F | Canary yellow | Latin | 486 |
| 1173 | Gustavo | M | Staff of the Goths | Italian/Spanish | 485 |
| 1174 | Leyla | F | Born at night | Arabic | 485 |
| 1175 | Jamari | M | | | 484 |
| 1176 | Jaylah | F | | | 484 |
| 1177 | Marvin | M | Lover of the sea | English | 483 |
| 1178 | Mauricio | M | Dark skinned | Spanish | 482 |
| 1179 | Anahi | F | | | 481 |
| 1180 | Ahmad | M | To praise | Arabic | 480 |
| 1181 | Mohammad | M | Praiseworthy | Arabic | 480 |
| 1182 | Jaliyah | F | | | 479 |
| 1183 | Justice | M | Just | Latin | 479 |
| 1184 | Kailani | F | | | 479 |

| 1185 | Trey | M | Three | Old English | 479 |
|------|------|---|-------|-------------|-----|
| 1186 | Elian | M | | | 478 |
| 1187 | Harlee | F | | | 477 |
| 1188 | Mohammed | M | Praiseworthy | Arabic | 477 |
| 1189 | Sincere | M | | | 477 |
| 1190 | Yusuf | M | God will add | Arabic | 477 |
| 1191 | Arturo | M | Noble | Italian | 475 |
| 1192 | Callen | M | | | 475 |
| 1193 | Rayan | M | | | 475 |
| 1194 | Wynter | F | | | 475 |
| 1195 | Saige | F | | | 474 |
| 1196 | Alessia | F | | | 473 |
| 1197 | Keaton | M | Where hawks fly | English | 473 |
| 1198 | Wilder | M | | | 472 |
| 1199 | Mekhi | M | | | 471 |
| 1200 | Memphis | M | | | 471 |
| 1201 | Cayson | M | | | 470 |
| 1202 | Monica | F | Advisor | Latin | 469 |
| 1203 | Anya | F | Grace form of Anna | Russian | 468 |
| 1204 | Antonella | F | | | 467 |
| 1205 | Emberly | F | | | 467 |
| 1206 | Conrad | M | Honest or brave advisor | German | 466 |
| 1207 | Khaleesi | F | | | 466 |
| 1208 | Kaison | M | | | 465 |
| 1209 | Kyree | M | | | 465 |
| 1210 | Ivory | F | Creamy white | Latin | 464 |
| 1211 | Soren | M | Stern or strict | Scandinavian | 464 |
| 1212 | Colby | M | From the dark farmstead | Old English | 463 |
| 1213 | Greta | F | Pearl | German | 463 |
| 1214 | Maren | F | Bitter or sea of bitterness | Arabic | 463 |
| 1215 | Alena | F | Fair | Celtic | 462 |
| 1216 | Bryant | M | Virtuous | Irish | 462 |
| 1217 | Emory | F | Industrious ruler | German | 462 |
| 1218 | Lucian | M | Bringer of light | Latin | 462 |
| 1219 | Alfredo | M | Wise counselor | Spanish | 461 |
| 1220 | Cassius | M | | | 461 |
| 1221 | Alaia | F | | | 460 |

| 1222 | Cynthia | F | Moon | Greek | 460 |
|---|---|---|---|---|---|
| 1223 | Marcelo | M | | | 460 |
| 1224 | Nikolas | M | | | 460 |
| 1225 | Addisyn | F | | | 459 |
| 1226 | Alia | F | | | 458 |
| 1227 | Brennan | M | Little raven | Irish | 458 |
| 1228 | Darren | M | Great | Irish | 457 |
| 1229 | Jasiah | M | | | 457 |
| 1230 | Lylah | F | | | 457 |
| 1231 | Angie | F | | | 456 |
| 1232 | Ariya | F | | | 456 |
| 1233 | Jimmy | M | Supplanted | English | 456 |
| 1234 | Lionel | M | Young lion | French | 456 |
| 1235 | Reece | M | Enthusiastic | Welsh | 456 |
| 1236 | Ty | M | Tile maker | English | 456 |
| 1237 | Alma | F | Soul | Latin | 455 |
| 1238 | Crystal | F | Clear or unblemished | Latin | 455 |
| 1239 | Jayde | F | Stone of the side | American | 455 |
| 1240 | Aileen | F | Light bearer | Irish | 454 |
| 1241 | Chris | M | Follower of Christ or anointed | Greek | 454 |
| 1242 | Forrest | M | Woodsman | French | 454 |
| 1243 | Kinslee | F | | | 454 |
| 1244 | Siena | F | | | 454 |
| 1245 | Zelda | F | Companion | Old English | 454 |
| 1246 | Katalina | F | | | 453 |
| 1247 | Korbin | M | Raven haired | English | 453 |
| 1248 | Marie | F | Bitter or sea of bitterness | French | 453 |
| 1249 | Pearl | F | Pearl | Latin | 453 |
| 1250 | Reyna | F | | | 453 |
| 1251 | Mae | F | Great | English | 452 |
| 1252 | Zahra | F | To blossom | Arabic | 452 |
| 1253 | Kailey | F | Laurel | American | 451 |
| 1254 | Jessie | F | He sees | Hebrew | 450 |
| 1255 | Tatum | M | Light hearted | English | 449 |
| 1256 | Tiana | F | | | 449 |
| 1257 | Amirah | F | Princess | Arabic | 448 |
| 1258 | Madalyn | F | From the high tower | Greek | 448 |

| 1259 | Jalen | M | Calm or serene | American | 447 |
|------|-------|---|----------------|----------|-----|
| 1260 | Alaya | F | | | 446 |
| 1261 | Santino | M | | | 444 |
| 1262 | Lilyana | F | | | 443 |
| 1263 | Julissa | F | | | 441 |
| 1264 | Case | M | Brave | Irish | 439 |
| 1265 | Armani | F | | | 438 |
| 1266 | Lennox | F | With many elm trees | Scottish | 438 |
| 1267 | Lillie | F | Lily | Latin | 438 |
| 1268 | Jolie | F | Pretty | French | 437 |
| 1269 | Laney | F | A narrow country road | Old English | 437 |
| 1270 | Roselyn | F | Red haired | French | 437 |
| 1271 | Mara | F | Eternally beautiful | Greek | 436 |
| 1272 | Joelle | F | God is willing | Hebrew | 435 |
| 1273 | Rosa | F | Rose | Spanish | 435 |
| 1274 | Kaylani | F | | | 434 |
| 1275 | Leonard | M | Brave as a lion | German | 434 |
| 1276 | Alvin | M | Noble friend | German | 432 |
| 1277 | Bridget | F | Strength | Irish | 432 |
| 1278 | Issac | M | | | 432 |
| 1279 | Liv | F | Life | Old Norse | 432 |
| 1280 | Oaklyn | F | | | 432 |
| 1281 | Aurelia | F | Gold | Latin | 431 |
| 1282 | Bo | M | Attractive | American | 431 |
| 1283 | Quincy | M | Fifth | French | 431 |
| 1284 | Clarissa | F | Bright or clear | Italian | 430 |
| 1285 | Mack | M | Son of | Celtic | 430 |
| 1286 | Samson | M | Bright sun | Hebrew | 430 |
| 1287 | Rex | M | | | 428 |
| 1288 | Alberto | M | Bright nobility | Italian | 427 |
| 1289 | Callum | M | Bald dove | Scottish | 427 |
| 1290 | Curtis | M | Polite or courteous | French | 427 |
| 1291 | Elyse | F | Noble | German | 427 |
| 1292 | Marissa | F | Of the sea | Latin | 427 |
| 1293 | Monroe | F | From the river's mouth | Irish | 427 |
| 1294 | Kori | F | | | 426 |
| 1295 | Hezekiah | M | God is my strength | Hebrew | 425 |

| | | | | | |
|------|----------|---|---------------------------|----------|-----|
| 1296 | Elsa | F | Noble | German | 424 |
| 1297 | Finnley | M | | | 424 |
| 1298 | Rosie | F | | | 424 |
| 1299 | Amelie | F | Hard working | French | 423 |
| 1300 | Aliza | F | Joy or delight | Hebrew | 422 |
| 1301 | Aitana | F | | | 422 |
| 1302 | Briggs | M | | | 422 |
| 1303 | Kamari | M | | | 422 |
| 1304 | Zeke | M | Strength of God | Hebrew | 422 |
| 1305 | Eileen | F | Light | Irish | 421 |
| 1306 | Poppy | F | Flower | Latin | 421 |
| 1307 | Emmie | F | | | 420 |
| 1308 | Raylan | M | | | 420 |
| 1309 | Neil | M | Champion | Irish | 419 |
| 1310 | Braylee | F | | | 418 |
| 1311 | Milana | F | | | 418 |
| 1312 | Titan | M | | | 418 |
| 1313 | Julien | M | Downy bearded or youthful | Latin | 417 |
| 1314 | Kellen | M | | | 417 |
| 1315 | Devon | M | Poet | Irish | 416 |
| 1316 | Addilynn | F | | | 415 |
| 1317 | Kylan | M | Land where cattle graze | Scottish | 415 |
| 1318 | Roger | M | Famous warrior | German | 415 |
| 1319 | Royal | F | Regal | French | 415 |
| 1320 | Axton | M | Swordsman's stone | English | 414 |
| 1321 | Chaya | F | Life | Hebrew | 414 |
| 1322 | Frida | F | | | 414 |
| 1323 | Bonnie | F | Pretty | English | 412 |
| 1324 | Amora | F | Love | Spanish | 411 |
| 1325 | Carl | M | Farmer | German | 411 |
| 1326 | Douglas | M | Dark stream or dark river | Scottish | 411 |
| 1327 | Larry | M | Crowned with laurels | Latin | 411 |
| 1328 | Stevie | F | Crown or wreath | Latin | 411 |
| 1329 | Crosby | M | | | 410 |
| 1330 | Tatiana | F | Fairy princess | Russian | 410 |
| 1331 | Malaya | F | | | 409 |
| 1332 | Mina | F | Love | German | 409 |

| 1333 | Fletcher | M | Arrow maker | Old English | 408 |
|------|----------|---|-------------|-------------|-----|
| 1334 | Emerie | F | | | 408 |
| 1335 | Makai | M | | | 408 |
| 1336 | Nelson | M | Son of Neil | English | 407 |
| 1337 | Reign | F | | | 407 |
| 1338 | Hamza | M | | | 406 |
| 1339 | Zaylee | F | | | 405 |
| 1340 | Annika | F | Gracious | Swedish | 404 |
| 1341 | Kenia | F | | | 404 |
| 1342 | Lance | M | Attendant | German | 404 |
| 1343 | Linda | F | Tender beauty | Spanish | 404 |
| 1344 | Alden | M | Old and wise protector | Old English | 403 |
| 1345 | Gary | M | Mighty with a spear | English | 403 |
| 1346 | Kenna | F | Beautiful | Irish | 403 |
| 1347 | Wilson | M | Son of William | English | 402 |
| 1348 | Alessandro | M | Defender of mankind | Italian | 401 |
| 1349 | Ares | M | | | 401 |
| 1350 | Faye | F | Trust or belief | English | 401 |
| 1351 | Kashton | M | | | 401 |
| 1352 | Reina | F | Queen | Latin | 401 |
| 1353 | Brittany | F | From Britain | Old English | 400 |
| 1354 | Bruno | M | Brown | German | 400 |
| 1355 | Jakob | M | Supplanted | German | 400 |
| 1356 | Marina | F | Sea maiden | Latin | 400 |
| 1357 | Astrid | F | Beautiful Goddess | Old Norse | 399 |
| 1358 | Kadence | F | | | 399 |
| 1359 | Mikaela | F | Who is like God | Hebrew | 399 |
| 1360 | Stetson | M | | | 399 |
| 1361 | Zain | M | God is Gracious | English | 399 |
| 1362 | Cairo | M | | | 398 |
| 1363 | Jaelyn | F | | | 398 |
| 1364 | Nathanael | M | Gift from God | Hebrew | 398 |
| 1365 | Byron | M | At the cowshed | Old English | 397 |
| 1366 | Briar | F | | | 397 |
| 1367 | Harry | M | Ruler of an enclosure | Old English | 397 |
| 1368 | Kaylie | F | Pure | American | 396 |
| 1369 | Harley | M | From yhe hare's meadow | English | 395 |

| 1370 | Mitchell | M | Who is like God | Old English | 395 |
|------|----------|---|-----------------|-------------|-----|
| 1371 | Teresa | F | Harvester | Greek | 395 |
| 1372 | Bria | F | Strong | Irish | 394 |
| 1373 | Maurice | M | Dark skinned | Latin | 394 |
| 1374 | Hadassah | F | Myrtle tree | Hebrew | 393 |
| 1375 | Lilianna | F | | | 393 |
| 1376 | Guadalupe | F | Valley of the wolf | Spanish | 391 |
| 1377 | Orlando | M | Renowned in the land | German | 391 |
| 1378 | Rayna | F | | | 391 |
| 1379 | Chanel | F | Chanel | English | 390 |
| 1380 | Kingsley | M | From the king's meadow | Old English | 390 |
| 1381 | Lyra | F | Expression of emotion | Greek | 390 |
| 1382 | Noa | F | | | 389 |
| 1383 | Zariyah | F | | | 389 |
| 1384 | Kaysen | M | | | 388 |
| 1385 | Laylah | F | | | 388 |
| 1386 | Sylas | M | | | 388 |
| 1387 | Trent | M | Gushing Waters | Latin | 388 |
| 1388 | Aubrielle | F | | | 386 |
| 1389 | Aniya | F | | | 385 |
| 1390 | Livia | F | Crown | Hebrew | 385 |
| 1391 | Ramon | M | Wisely | Spanish | 385 |
| 1392 | Boston | M | | | 384 |
| 1393 | Lucca | M | | | 384 |
| 1394 | Noe | M | Rest or comfort | French | 384 |
| 1395 | Ellen | F | Light | English | 383 |
| 1396 | Meadow | F | A clearing | Old English | 383 |
| 1397 | Jagger | M | Hunter | German | 382 |
| 1398 | Reyansh | M | | | 382 |
| 1399 | Vihaan | M | | | 382 |
| 1400 | Randy | M | Wolf's shield | English | 381 |
| 1401 | Amiya | F | | | 380 |
| 1402 | Ellis | F | The Lord is my God | English | 380 |
| 1403 | Elora | F | God is light | Unknown | 380 |
| 1404 | Milan | F | | | 380 |
| 1405 | Thaddeus | M | Wise | Greek | 380 |
| 1406 | Hunter | F | A huntsman | English | 379 |

| 1407 | Lennon | M | Small cloak or cape | Irish | 379 |
|---|---|---|---|---|---|
| 1408 | Princess | F | Daughter of royalty | Old English | 379 |
| 1409 | Leanna | F | Meadow | Old English | 378 |
| 1410 | Nathalie | F | Birthday of Christ | Russian | 378 |
| 1411 | Clementine | F | Merciful | Latin | 377 |
| 1412 | Kannon | M | | | 376 |
| 1413 | Kohen | M | | | 376 |
| 1414 | Tristen | M | Bold | Welsh | 375 |
| 1415 | Valentino | M | Healthy or strong | Latin | 375 |
| 1416 | Maxton | M | | | 374 |
| 1417 | Nola | F | Famous | Celtic | 374 |
| 1418 | Salvador | M | Savior | Spanish | 374 |
| 1419 | Tenley | F | | | 374 |
| 1420 | Abdiel | M | | | 373 |
| 1421 | Langston | M | From the long enclosure | English | 373 |
| 1422 | Simone | F | Heard | Hebrew | 373 |
| 1423 | Lina | F | Light | Greek | 372 |
| 1424 | Rohan | M | Red haired | Irish | 371 |
| 1425 | Kristopher | M | | | 370 |
| 1426 | Marianna | F | War like | Latin | 370 |
| 1427 | Martha | F | Sorrow | Arabic | 370 |
| 1428 | Sariah | F | | | 370 |
| 1429 | Louisa | F | Famous warrior | English | 369 |
| 1430 | Noemi | F | Pleasantness | Hebrew | 369 |
| 1431 | Emmeline | F | Industrious | French | 368 |
| 1432 | Kenley | F | From the king's meadow | English | 368 |
| 1433 | Belen | F | Bethlehem | Unknown | 367 |
| 1434 | Yosef | M | God will add | Hebrew | 366 |
| 1435 | Erika | F | Eternal ruler | Old Norse | 365 |
| 1436 | Rayden | M | | | 365 |
| 1437 | Lee | M | Dweller near the wood or clearing | Old English | 364 |
| 1438 | Myah | F | | | 364 |
| 1439 | Callan | M | | | 363 |
| 1440 | Lara | F | Cheerful | Greek | 363 |
| 1441 | Tripp | M | Traveler | English | 363 |
| 1442 | Ansley | F | My own meadow | English | 362 |
| 1443 | Amani | F | | | 362 |

| 1444 | Deandre | M | Strong and womanly | American | 362 |
|------|---------|---|--------------------|----------|-----|
| 1445 | Everlee | F | | | 362 |
| 1446 | Joe | M | God will add | Hebrew | 362 |
| 1447 | Maleah | F | | | 362 |
| 1448 | Morgan | M | Bright Sea | Welsh | 362 |
| 1449 | Salma | F | Safe | Arabic | 361 |
| 1450 | Dariel | M | Little darling | French | 360 |
| 1451 | Colten | M | Coal town | Old English | 358 |
| 1452 | Jaelynn | F | | | 358 |
| 1453 | Reese | M | Ardor | Welsh | 358 |
| 1454 | Jedidiah | M | Friend of God or beloved of God | Hebrew | 357 |
| 1455 | Ricky | M | Powerful ruler | German | 357 |
| 1456 | Kiera | F | Dark haired one | Irish | 356 |
| 1457 | Dulce | F | Sweet | Spanish | 355 |
| 1458 | Nala | F | | | 355 |
| 1459 | Natasha | F | Born at Christmas | Russian | 355 |
| 1460 | Bronson | M | Son of the dark man | English | 354 |
| 1461 | Averi | F | | | 354 |
| 1462 | Mercy | F | Compassion | English | 354 |
| 1463 | Penny | F | Bobbin worker | Greek | 354 |
| 1464 | Terry | M | Harvester | Greek | 354 |
| 1465 | Ariadne | F | | | 353 |
| 1466 | Deborah | F | Bee | Hebrew | 353 |
| 1467 | Eddie | M | Names beginning with Ed | English | 353 |
| 1468 | Elisabeth | F | God is my oath | Hebrew | 353 |
| 1469 | Jefferson | M | Son of Jeff | Old English | 353 |
| 1470 | Lachlan | M | From the land of lakes | Scottish | 353 |
| 1471 | Layne | M | A narrow country road | Old English | 353 |
| 1472 | Zaria | F | Blossom | Arabic | 353 |
| 1473 | Clay | M | Settlement by the clay pit | Old English | 352 |
| 1474 | Hana | F | | | 352 |
| 1475 | Kairi | F | | | 352 |
| 1476 | Madden | M | Small dog Milos | Unknown | 352 |
| 1477 | Yareli | F | | | 352 |
| 1478 | Jamir | M | | | 351 |
| 1479 | Raina | F | Queen | Latin | 351 |

| 1480 | Tomas | M | Twin | German | 351 |
|---|---|---|---|---|---|
| 1481 | Ryann | F | Little ruler | Irish | 349 |
| 1482 | Kareem | M | Generous | Arabic | 348 |
| 1483 | Lexie | F | Defender of mankind | Greek | 348 |
| 1484 | Stanley | M | Lives by the stony meadow | Old English | 348 |
| 1485 | Thalia | F | | | 348 |
| 1486 | Karter | F | | | 347 |
| 1487 | Annabel | F | Beautiful grace | Old English | 346 |
| 1488 | Christine | F | Follower of Christ or anointed | Greek | 346 |
| 1489 | Estella | F | Star | Spanish | 346 |
| 1490 | Brayan | M | | | 346 |
| 1491 | Amos | M | Burden | Hebrew | 345 |
| 1492 | Kase | M | | | 345 |
| 1493 | Keyla | F | | | 345 |
| 1494 | Kristian | M | | | 345 |
| 1495 | Adele | F | Noble | English | 344 |
| 1496 | Aya | F | Bird | Hebrew | 344 |
| 1497 | Clyde | M | Warm or refers the Clyde river | Scottish | 344 |
| 1498 | Ernesto | M | Sincere | Spanish | 344 |
| 1499 | Estelle | F | Star | French | 344 |
| 1500 | Landry | F | Ruler | Old English | 344 |
| 1501 | Tommy | M | Twin | English | 344 |
| 1502 | Tori | F | Triumphant | Old English | 344 |
| 1503 | Perla | F | Pearl | Latin | 343 |
| 1504 | Lailah | F | | | 342 |
| 1505 | Miah | F | | | 342 |
| 1506 | Casen | M | | | 341 |
| 1507 | Rylan | F | Island meadow | Irish | 341 |
| 1508 | Angelique | F | Messenger of God | French | 340 |
| 1509 | Avalynn | F | | | 340 |
| 1510 | Ford | M | River crossing | Old English | 340 |
| 1511 | Crew | M | | | 339 |
| 1512 | Romina | F | | | 339 |
| 1513 | Braydon | M | Broad valley | Old English | 338 |
| 1514 | Ari | F | Lion | Hebrew | 337 |
| 1515 | Brecken | M | | | 337 |

| 1516 | Jaycee | F | Attractive | Greek | 337 |
|------|--------|---|------------|-------|-----|
| 1517 | Hassan | M | Handsome | Arabic | 336 |
| 1518 | Jaylene | F | Jaybird | American | 336 |
| 1519 | Kai | F | Earth | Greek | 336 |
| 1520 | Louise | F | Famous warrior | German | 336 |
| 1521 | Mavis | F | Joy | French | 336 |
| 1522 | Scarlette | F | | | 336 |
| 1523 | Belle | F | Beautiful | French | 335 |
| 1524 | Axl | M | | | 335 |
| 1525 | Lea | F | Tired or weary | Hebrew | 335 |
| 1526 | Nalani | F | | | 335 |
| 1527 | Rivka | F | Captivating | Hebrew | 335 |
| 1528 | Boone | M | Good | Latin | 334 |
| 1529 | Ayleen | F | | | 334 |
| 1530 | Calliope | F | | | 334 |
| 1531 | Dalary | F | | | 334 |
| 1532 | Zaniyah | F | | | 334 |
| 1533 | Leandro | M | Lion man or brave as a lion | Spanish | 333 |
| 1534 | Samir | M | | | 333 |
| 1535 | Jaziel | M | | | 332 |
| 1536 | Kaelyn | F | Sweetheart | Hebrew | 332 |
| 1537 | Sky | F | | | 332 |
| 1538 | Jewel | F | Rare excellence | Latin | 331 |
| 1539 | Magnus | M | Great | Latin | 331 |
| 1540 | Abdullah | M | Servant of God | Arabic | 330 |
| 1541 | Joselyn | F | | | 330 |
| 1542 | Madalynn | F | From the high tower | Greek | 330 |
| 1543 | Paola | F | Little | Latin | 330 |
| 1544 | Yousef | M | | | 330 |
| 1545 | Giovanna | F | God is gracious | Italian | 329 |
| 1546 | Isabela | F | Consecrated to God | Spanish | 328 |
| 1547 | Karlee | F | Tiny and feminine | Latin | 328 |
| 1548 | Branson | M | Son of Brandon | Old English | 327 |
| 1549 | Aubriella | F | | | 327 |
| 1550 | Azariah | F | | | 327 |
| 1551 | Jadiel | M | | | 327 |
| 1552 | Jaxen | M | | | 327 |

| 1553 | Layton | M | From the meadow farm | English | 327 |
|---|---|---|---|---|---|
| 1554 | Tinley | F | | | 327 |
| 1555 | Franco | M | Free or form France | Spanish | 326 |
| 1556 | Dream | F | | | 326 |
| 1557 | Ben | M | Born of the right hand | Hebrew | 325 |
| 1558 | Claudia | F | Lame | Latin | 325 |
| 1559 | Corinne | F | Maiden | Greek | 325 |
| 1560 | Erica | F | Eternal ruler | Scandinavian | 325 |
| 1561 | Grey | M | Gray haired | English | 325 |
| 1562 | Kelvin | M | From the narrow river or river man | Old English | 325 |
| 1563 | Milena | F | | | 325 |
| 1564 | Aliana | F | | | 324 |
| 1565 | Kallie | F | Most beautiful | Greek | 324 |
| 1566 | Alyson | F | Truthful | Old English | 323 |
| 1567 | Chaim | M | Life | Hebrew | 323 |
| 1568 | Demetrius | M | Of the earth | Greek | 323 |
| 1569 | Joyce | F | Rejoicing | Latin | 323 |
| 1570 | Tinsley | F | | | 323 |
| 1571 | Whitney | F | White island | Old English | 323 |
| 1572 | Blaine | M | Slender or thin | Irish | 322 |
| 1573 | Emilee | F | | | 322 |
| 1574 | Paisleigh | F | | | 322 |
| 1575 | Ridge | M | From the ridge | English | 322 |
| 1576 | Carolyn | F | Little and womanly | English | 321 |
| 1577 | Colson | M | Victory of the people | English | 321 |
| 1578 | Jaylee | F | | | 321 |
| 1579 | Melvin | M | Council or protector | Old English | 321 |
| 1580 | Zoie | F | | | 321 |
| 1581 | Anakin | M | | | 320 |
| 1582 | Aryan | M | | | 320 |
| 1583 | Frankie | F | Free or from France | American | 320 |
| 1584 | Andi | F | Courageous | American | 319 |
| 1585 | Judith | F | From Judea | Hebrew | 319 |
| 1586 | Lochlan | M | | | 319 |
| 1587 | Paula | F | Small | Latin | 319 |
| 1588 | Xiomara | F | | | 319 |
| 1589 | Aiyana | F | Eternal blossom | Unknown | 318 |

| 1590 | Amia | F | Beloved | French | 318 |
|---|---|---|---|---|---|
| 1591 | Audrina | F | Noble strength | Old English | 318 |
| 1592 | Analia | F | | | 318 |
| 1593 | Hadlee | F | | | 318 |
| 1594 | Jon | M | God is gracious | Hebrew | 318 |
| 1595 | Rayne | F | Strong counselor | English | 318 |
| 1596 | Amayah | F | | | 317 |
| 1597 | Cara | F | Dear or beloved | Latin | 317 |
| 1598 | Celia | F | Blind | Latin | 317 |
| 1599 | Canaan | M | | | 317 |
| 1600 | Dash | M | | | 317 |
| 1601 | Lyanna | F | | | 317 |
| 1602 | Opal | F | Precious stone | Hindi | 317 |
| 1603 | Zechariah | M | Jehovah has remembered | Hebrew | 317 |
| 1604 | Alonso | M | Eager for battle | Spanish | 316 |
| 1605 | Amaris | F | Given by God | Hebrew | 316 |
| 1606 | Otis | M | Wealthy | German | 316 |
| 1607 | Zaire | M | | | 316 |
| 1608 | Clare | F | Bright or Clear | Latin | 315 |
| 1609 | Gwen | F | White wave | Welsh | 315 |
| 1610 | Giana | F | | | 314 |
| 1611 | Marcel | M | Warlike | French | 314 |
| 1612 | Veda | F | | | 314 |
| 1613 | Alisha | F | | | 313 |
| 1614 | Davina | F | Beloved | Scottish | 313 |
| 1615 | Rhea | F | Flowing | Greek | 313 |
| 1616 | Sariyah | F | | | 313 |
| 1617 | Brett | M | From Britain | Irish | 312 |
| 1618 | Stefan | M | Crowned or crown of laurels | Hebrew | 312 |
| 1619 | Aldo | M | Old or wise | Italian | 311 |
| 1620 | Jeffery | M | Divinely peaceful | Old English | 311 |
| 1621 | Noor | F | | | 311 |
| 1622 | Baylor | M | | | 310 |
| 1623 | Danica | F | | | 310 |
| 1624 | Kathleen | F | Pure | Irish | 310 |
| 1625 | Lillianna | F | | | 310 |

| 1626 | Lindsey | F | Island of linden trees | Old English | 310 |
|------|---------|---|------------------------|-------------|-----|
| 1627 | Talon | M | Claw | English | 310 |
| 1628 | Dominik | M | Belonging to the Lord | Polish | 309 |
| 1629 | Flynn | M | Son of a red-haired man | Irish | 309 |
| 1630 | Maxine | F | The greatest | Latin | 309 |
| 1631 | Paulina | F | Small | Latin | 309 |
| 1632 | Carmelo | M | Fruitful orchard | Hebrew | 308 |
| 1633 | Dane | M | From Denmark | Old English | 308 |
| 1634 | Harleigh | F | From the hare's meadow | English | 308 |
| 1635 | Jamal | M | Handsome | Arabic | 308 |
| 1636 | Hailee | F | | | 308 |
| 1637 | Kole | M | | | 308 |
| 1638 | Nancy | F | Full of grace | English | 308 |
| 1639 | Enoch | M | Consecrated or dedicated | Hebrew | 307 |
| 1640 | Jessa | F | | | 307 |
| 1641 | Raquel | F | Innocence of a lamb | Latin | 307 |
| 1642 | Raylee | F | | | 307 |
| 1643 | Zainab | F | | | 307 |
| 1644 | Chana | F | Graceful | Hebrew | 306 |
| 1645 | Graysen | M | Son of the gray-haired man | Old English | 306 |
| 1646 | Kye | M | Land where cattle graze | Scottish | 305 |
| 1647 | Lisa | F | Consecrated to God | Hebrew | 305 |
| 1648 | Vicente | M | Conqueror | Spanish | 305 |
| 1649 | Fisher | M | | | 304 |
| 1650 | Heavenly | F | | | 304 |
| 1651 | Oaklynn | F | | | 304 |
| 1652 | Ray | M | Regal | French | 304 |
| 1653 | Aminah | F | Trustworthy | Arabic | 303 |
| 1654 | Fox | M | | | 303 |
| 1655 | Jamie | M | Supplanted | English | 302 |
| 1656 | Emmalynn | F | | | 302 |
| 1657 | Patricia | F | Noble | Latin | 302 |
| 1658 | Rey | M | Kingly | Spanish | 302 |
| 1659 | Zaid | M | | | 302 |
| 1660 | Allan | M | Handsome | Irish | 301 |
| 1661 | Emery | M | Industrious ruler | German | 301 |

| 1662 | Gannon | M | Light skinned | Irish | 301 |
|------|--------|---|---------------|-------|-----|
| 1663 | Joziah | M | Jehovah has healed | Unknown | 301 |
| 1664 | Rodney | M | Island clearing | English | 301 |
| 1665 | India | F | River | Unknown | 300 |
| 1666 | Janessa | F | | | 300 |
| 1667 | Juelz | M | | | 300 |
| 1668 | Sonny | M | A young boy | English | 300 |
| 1669 | Terrance | M | Smooth | Latin | 300 |
| 1670 | Zyaire | M | | | 300 |
| 1671 | Augustine | M | Majestic | Latin | 299 |
| 1672 | Cory | M | Dweller near a hollow | Irish | 299 |
| 1673 | Paloma | F | Dove | Spanish | 299 |
| 1674 | Ramona | F | Wise protector | Spanish | 299 |
| 1675 | Sandra | F | Defender of mankind | Greek | 299 |
| 1676 | Felipe | M | Lover of horses | Spanish | 298 |
| 1677 | Abril | F | Second | Spanish | 297 |
| 1678 | Aron | M | Lofty or inspired | Hebrew | 297 |
| 1679 | Emmaline | F | Industrious | French | 297 |
| 1680 | Itzayana | F | | | 297 |
| 1681 | Jacoby | M | | | 297 |
| 1682 | Kassandra | F | | | 297 |
| 1683 | Vienna | F | | | 297 |
| 1684 | Harlan | M | From the hare's land | English | 296 |
| 1685 | Marc | M | Warlike | French | 296 |
| 1686 | Marleigh | F | From the lake meadow | English | 296 |
| 1687 | Bobby | M | Bright fame | English | 295 |
| 1688 | Joey | M | God will add | Hebrew | 295 |
| 1689 | Kailyn | F | Laurel | American | 294 |
| 1690 | Novalee | F | | | 294 |
| 1691 | Rosalyn | F | | | 294 |
| 1692 | Anson | M | Anne's son | English | 293 |
| 1693 | Hadleigh | F | | | 293 |
| 1694 | Luella | F | Famous elf | English | 293 |
| 1695 | Taliyah | F | | | 293 |
| 1696 | Barbara | F | Foreign or stranger | Latin | 292 |
| 1697 | Avalyn | F | | | 292 |
| 1698 | Iliana | F | Light | Greek | 292 |

| 1699 | Jana | F | God is gracious | Slavic | 292 |
|---|---|---|---|---|---|
| 1700 | Meilani | F | | | 292 |
| 1701 | Aadhya | F | | | 290 |
| 1702 | Alannah | F | Attractive | Irish | 290 |
| 1703 | Blaire | F | Dweller on the plain | Scottish | 290 |
| 1704 | Brenda | F | Little raven | Irish | 290 |
| 1705 | Casey | F | Brave | Irish | 290 |
| 1706 | Huxley | M | From Hugh's meadow | Old English | 290 |
| 1707 | Marlon | M | Falcon | French | 290 |
| 1708 | Anders | M | Manly | Scandinavian | 289 |
| 1709 | Selene | F | | | 289 |
| 1710 | Lizbeth | F | Consecrated to God | English | 288 |
| 1711 | Adrienne | F | Dark | Latin | 287 |
| 1712 | Annalee | F | Gracious | English | 287 |
| 1713 | Guillermo | M | Resolute protector | Spanish | 287 |
| 1714 | Malani | F | | | 287 |
| 1715 | Payton | M | Noble woman | Irish | 287 |
| 1716 | Castiel | M | | | 286 |
| 1717 | Damari | M | | | 286 |
| 1718 | Shepherd | M | Shepherd | English | 286 |
| 1719 | Aliya | F | | | 285 |
| 1720 | Azariah | M | | | 285 |
| 1721 | Harold | M | Ruler of the army | Old Norse | 285 |
| 1722 | Miley | F | | | 285 |
| 1723 | Nataly | F | | | 285 |
| 1724 | Bexley | F | | | 284 |
| 1725 | Harper | M | Harpist or minstrel | English | 284 |
| 1726 | Joslyn | F | Joyous | Latin | 284 |
| 1727 | Maliah | F | | | 284 |
| 1728 | Zion | F | Sign | Hebrew | 284 |
| 1729 | Breanna | F | Virtuous | Irish | 283 |
| 1730 | Henrik | M | Ruler of the enclosure | Dutch | 283 |
| 1731 | Houston | M | Hill town | Old English | 283 |
| 1732 | Melania | F | Dark or black | Greek | 283 |
| 1733 | Estrella | F | Star | Spanish | 282 |
| 1734 | Kairo | M | | | 282 |
| 1735 | Ingrid | F | Beautiful or fair | Old Norse | 281 |

| 1736 | Jayden | F | Jade | American | 281 |
|------|--------|---|------|----------|-----|
| 1737 | Kaya | F | | | 281 |
| 1738 | Kaylin | F | Pure | American | 281 |
| 1739 | Willie | M | Resolute protector | German | 281 |
| 1740 | Elisha | M | God is my salvation | Hebrew | 280 |
| 1741 | Harmoni | F | | | 280 |
| 1742 | Ameer | M | | | 279 |
| 1743 | Arely | F | | | 279 |
| 1744 | Jazlynn | F | Fragrant flower | American | 279 |
| 1745 | Kiana | F | Favored grace | Hawaiian | 279 |
| 1746 | Dana | F | From Denmark | Old Norse | 278 |
| 1747 | Emory | M | Industrious ruler | German | 278 |
| 1748 | Mylah | F | | | 278 |
| 1749 | Oaklee | F | | | 278 |
| 1750 | Skylar | M | The isle of Skye | Scottish | 278 |
| 1751 | Ailani | F | | | 277 |
| 1752 | Kailee | F | Laurel | American | 277 |
| 1753 | Legacy | F | | | 277 |
| 1754 | Marjorie | F | | | 277 |
| 1755 | Paityn | F | | | 277 |
| 1756 | Sutton | M | From the south farm | English | 277 |
| 1757 | Alfonso | M | Noble and eager | Italian | 276 |
| 1758 | Brentley | M | Hilltop | English | 276 |
| 1759 | Courtney | F | Courtier or court attendant | English | 276 |
| 1760 | Ellianna | F | | | 276 |
| 1761 | Jurnee | F | | | 276 |
| 1762 | Karlie | F | Tiny and feminine | Latin | 276 |
| 1763 | Toby | M | The Lord is good | Hebrew | 276 |
| 1764 | Evalyn | F | Hazelnut | Old English | 275 |
| 1765 | Holland | F | | | 275 |
| 1766 | Kenya | F | Animal horn | Hebrew | 275 |
| 1767 | Magdalena | F | From the high tower | Spanish | 275 |
| 1768 | Blaze | M | Stammered | Latin | 274 |
| 1769 | Carla | F | Little and womanly | English | 274 |
| 1770 | Eugene | M | Well born or noble | French | 274 |
| 1771 | Halle | F | Heroine | Scandinavian | 274 |
| 1772 | Shiloh | M | God's Gift | Hebrew | 274 |

| 1773 | Wayne | M | Wagon | Old English | 274 |
|---|---|---|---|---|---|
| 1774 | Aryanna | F | | | 273 |
| 1775 | Darian | M | Great | Irish | 273 |
| 1776 | Gordon | M | Hill near the meadow | Old English | 273 |
| 1777 | London | M | Fortress | Old English | 273 |
| 1778 | Bodie | M | | | 272 |
| 1779 | Jordy | M | To flow down or descend | Hebrew | 272 |
| 1780 | Kaiya | F | | | 272 |
| 1781 | Kimora | F | | | 272 |
| 1782 | Naya | F | | | 272 |
| 1783 | Saoirse | F | | | 272 |
| 1784 | Susan | F | Lily | Hebrew | 272 |
| 1785 | Desiree | F | Desired or longed for | French | 271 |
| 1786 | Ensley | F | | | 271 |
| 1787 | Jermaine | M | Brotherly | French | 271 |
| 1788 | Renee | F | Reborn | French | 271 |
| 1789 | Denver | M | Green valley | English | 270 |
| 1790 | Esperanza | F | Hope | Spanish | 270 |
| 1791 | Gerald | M | Mighty with a spear | German | 269 |
| 1792 | Merrick | M | | | 269 |
| 1793 | Treasure | F | | | 269 |
| 1794 | Ellison | F | Son of Elder | English | 268 |
| 1795 | Caylee | F | | | 268 |
| 1796 | Kristina | F | Follower of Christ | Greek | 268 |
| 1797 | Musa | M | Arabic form of Moses | Unknown | 268 |
| 1798 | Vincenzo | M | Conqueror | Italian | 268 |
| 1799 | Kody | M | | | 267 |
| 1800 | Yahir | M | | | 267 |
| 1801 | Adilynn | F | | | 266 |
| 1802 | Anabelle | F | | | 266 |
| 1803 | Egypt | F | Unknown | Unknown | 266 |
| 1804 | Spencer | F | Dispenser of provisions | Old English | 266 |
| 1805 | Tegan | F | Attractive | Welsh | 266 |
| 1806 | Brodie | M | A ditch | Scottish | 265 |
| 1807 | Aranza | F | | | 265 |
| 1808 | Trace | M | Fighter | Irish | 265 |
| 1809 | Vada | F | | | 265 |

| 1810 | Darwin | M | Dear friend | English | 264 |
|------|--------|---|-------------|---------|-----|
| 1811 | Emerald | F | Bright green | French | 264 |
| 1812 | Florence | F | Blooming or flowering | Latin | 264 |
| 1813 | Marlowe | F | Bitter | English | 264 |
| 1814 | Micah | F | Who is like God | Hebrew | 264 |
| 1815 | Sonia | F | | | 264 |
| 1816 | Sunny | F | Bright or cheerful | English | 264 |
| 1817 | Tadeo | M | Praise | Arabic | 264 |
| 1818 | Tara | F | Hill | Irish | 264 |
| 1819 | Billy | M | Resolute protector | Old English | 263 |
| 1820 | Bentlee | M | | | 263 |
| 1821 | Hugh | M | Bright mind | English | 263 |
| 1822 | Reginald | M | Powerful ruler | English | 263 |
| 1823 | Vance | M | Marshland | Old English | 263 |
| 1824 | Westin | M | West town | English | 263 |
| 1825 | Cain | M | Gatherer | Hebrew | 262 |
| 1826 | Riya | F | | | 262 |
| 1827 | Yara | F | | | 262 |
| 1828 | Alisa | F | Of the nobility | Greek | 261 |
| 1829 | Arian | M | Enchanted | Greek | 261 |
| 1830 | Dayton | M | Sunny town | Old English | 261 |
| 1831 | Javion | M | | | 261 |
| 1832 | Nathalia | F | Birthday of Christ | Russian | 261 |
| 1833 | Terrence | M | Smooth | Latin | 261 |
| 1834 | Yamileth | F | | | 261 |
| 1835 | Brysen | M | | | 260 |
| 1836 | Saanvi | F | | | 260 |
| 1837 | Samira | F | | | 260 |
| 1838 | Sylvie | F | Of the woods | Latin | 260 |
| 1839 | Brenna | F | Little raven | Irish | 259 |
| 1840 | Carlee | F | | | 259 |
| 1841 | Jaxxon | M | | | 259 |
| 1842 | Jenny | F | White wave | Welsh | 259 |
| 1843 | Thatcher | M | Roofer | English | 259 |
| 1844 | Landry | M | Ruler | Old English | 258 |
| 1845 | Miya | F | | | 258 |
| 1846 | Monserrat | F | | | 258 |

| 1847 | Zendaya | F | | | 258 |
|------|---------|---|---|---|-----|
| 1848 | Alora | F | | | 257 |
| 1849 | Bryleigh | F | | | 257 |
| 1850 | Rene | M | Reborn | French | 257 |
| 1851 | Westley | M | From the west meadow | English | 257 |
| 1852 | Winnie | F | White or fair | Celtic | 257 |
| 1853 | Alisson | F | | | 256 |
| 1854 | Aubri | F | | | 256 |
| 1855 | Miller | M | One who grinds grain | English | 256 |
| 1856 | Violeta | F | | | 256 |
| 1857 | Alvaro | M | Elf army | Spanish | 255 |
| 1858 | Cristiano | M | Follower of Christ or anointed | Spanish | 255 |
| 1859 | Dalia | F | Branch | Hebrew | 255 |
| 1860 | Eliseo | M | God is my salvation | Italian/Spanish | 255 |
| 1861 | Etta | F | Ruler of the home | Old English | 255 |
| 1862 | Rilynn | F | | | 255 |
| 1863 | Waverly | F | | | 255 |
| 1864 | Whitley | F | White meadow | Old English | 255 |
| 1865 | August | F | Venerable | Latin | 254 |
| 1866 | Ephraim | M | Doubly fruitful | Hebrew | 254 |
| 1867 | Emmarie | F | | | 254 |
| 1868 | Kaylynn | F | Pure | American | 254 |
| 1869 | Adrien | M | Dark | Latin | 253 |
| 1870 | Jerome | M | Holy name | Latin | 253 |
| 1871 | Khalid | M | Eternal | Arabic | 253 |
| 1872 | Luz | F | Light | Spanish | 253 |
| 1873 | Rosalee | F | | | 253 |
| 1874 | Abrielle | F | | | 252 |
| 1875 | Antonia | F | Priceless, inestimable or praiseworthy | Latin | 252 |
| 1876 | Aydin | M | | | 252 |
| 1877 | Farrah | F | Beautiful | English | 252 |
| 1878 | Kamari | F | | | 252 |
| 1879 | Mayson | M | | | 252 |
| 1880 | Robin | F | Bright fame | English | 252 |
| 1881 | Amaia | F | End | Basque | 251 |
| 1882 | Ann | F | Gracious | English | 251 |

| 1883 | Azaria | F | God helps | Hebrew | 251 |
|---|---|---|---|---|---|
| 1884 | Alyvia | F | | | 251 |
| 1885 | Elodie | F | | | 251 |
| 1886 | Scout | F | To observe or spy | Unknown | 251 |
| 1887 | Yasmin | F | Sweet smelling | Arabic | 251 |
| 1888 | Alfred | M | Wise counselor | Old English | 250 |
| 1889 | Asia | F | Sunrise | English | 250 |
| 1890 | Duncan | M | Brown warrior | Scottish | 250 |
| 1891 | Cherish | F | | | 250 |
| 1892 | Junior | M | Younger | Latin | 250 |
| 1893 | Kendall | M | Valley of the river Kent | Old English | 250 |
| 1894 | Marisol | F | Sunny sea | Spanish | 250 |
| 1895 | Zavier | M | | | 250 |
| 1896 | Koda | M | | | 249 |
| 1897 | Maison | M | | | 249 |
| 1898 | Raya | F | Friend | Hebrew | 249 |
| 1899 | Akira | F | Anchor | Unknown | 248 |
| 1900 | Della | F | Bright | German | 248 |
| 1901 | Eleanora | F | Light | Greek | 248 |
| 1902 | Emilie | F | Industrious | English | 248 |
| 1903 | Caspian | M | | | 248 |
| 1904 | Maxim | M | | | 248 |
| 1905 | Sarahi | F | | | 248 |
| 1906 | Bellamy | F | Beautiful Friend | Latin | 247 |
| 1907 | Kace | M | | | 247 |
| 1908 | Zackary | M | God remembers | Hebrew | 247 |
| 1909 | Chandler | F | Maker of candles | Old English | 246 |
| 1910 | Jaylynn | F | Jaybird | American | 246 |
| 1911 | Madyson | F | | | 246 |
| 1912 | Mariyah | F | | | 246 |
| 1913 | Palmer | F | Bearing a palm branch | English | 246 |
| 1914 | Rudy | M | Famous wolf | English | 246 |
| 1915 | Coleman | M | Dark skinned or coal miner | Old English | 245 |
| 1916 | Kamiyah | F | | | 245 |
| 1917 | Keagan | M | Fire | English | 245 |
| 1918 | Kolten | M | Coal town | English | 245 |
| 1919 | Maximo | M | | | 245 |

| 1920 | Montserrat | F | | | 245 |
|------|-----------|---|---|---|-----|
| 1921 | Anabella | F | | | 244 |
| 1922 | Dario | M | Affluent or wealthy | Spanish | 244 |
| 1923 | Davion | M | Brilliant Finn | American | 244 |
| 1924 | Kalel | M | | | 244 |
| 1925 | Malayah | F | | | 244 |
| 1926 | Saniyah | F | | | 244 |
| 1927 | Dani | F | God is my judge | Hebrew | 243 |
| 1928 | Briar | M | | | 243 |
| 1929 | Jairo | M | God enlightens | Spanish | 243 |
| 1930 | Misael | M | | | 243 |
| 1931 | Rogelio | M | Famous warrior | Spanish | 243 |
| 1932 | Sharon | F | Desert plain | Hebrew | 243 |
| 1933 | Terrell | M | Thunder ruler | German | 243 |
| 1934 | Raylynn | F | | | 242 |
| 1935 | Sally | F | Princess | English | 242 |
| 1936 | Addalyn | F | | | 241 |
| 1937 | Aubrianna | F | | | 241 |
| 1938 | Heath | M | A heath or a moor | Old English | 241 |
| 1939 | Giavanna | F | | | 241 |
| 1940 | Kensington | F | | | 241 |
| 1941 | Micheal | M | Who is like God | Hebrew | 241 |
| 1942 | Sailor | F | | | 241 |
| 1943 | Wesson | M | | | 241 |
| 1944 | Aaden | M | | | 240 |
| 1945 | Alianna | F | | | 240 |
| 1946 | Ciara | F | Black like a raven | Irish | 240 |
| 1947 | Brixton | M | | | 240 |
| 1948 | Draven | M | | | 240 |
| 1949 | Mollie | F | Bitter | Irish | 240 |
| 1950 | Xzavier | M | | | 240 |
| 1951 | Darrell | M | Darling | French | 239 |
| 1952 | Mercedes | F | Mercy or merciful | Spanish | 239 |
| 1953 | Micaela | F | Who is like God | Hebrew | 239 |
| 1954 | Nailah | F | One who succeeds | Arabic, North Africa | 239 |
| 1955 | Promise | F | | | 239 |
| 1956 | Shayla | F | Fairy palace | Irish | 239 |

| 1957 | Tabitha | F | Gazelle | Arabic | 239 |
|------|---------|---|---------|--------|-----|
| 1958 | Keanu | M | | | 238 |
| 1959 | Mattie | F | Mighty battle maiden | English | 238 |
| 1960 | Moriah | F | Jehovah is my teacher | Hebrew | 238 |
| 1961 | Ronnie | M | Rules with good judgment | Scottish | 238 |
| 1962 | Konnor | M | | | 237 |
| 1963 | Libby | F | Consecrated to God | Hebrew | 237 |
| 1964 | Lincoln | F | Settlement by the pool | Old English | 237 |
| 1965 | Will | M | Resolute protector | English | 237 |
| 1966 | Audriana | F | Noble strength | Old English | 236 |
| 1967 | Frankie | M | Free or from France | American | 236 |
| 1968 | Dangelo | M | | | 236 |
| 1969 | Kamilah | F | Perfection | Arabic | 236 |
| 1970 | Kamryn | M | Crooked nose | American | 236 |
| 1971 | Lilyanna | F | | | 236 |
| 1972 | Salvatore | M | Savior | Italian | 236 |
| 1973 | Santana | M | | | 236 |
| 1974 | Shaun | M | God is gracious | Irish | 236 |
| 1975 | Zola | F | | | 236 |
| 1976 | Aimee | F | Dearly loved | French | 235 |
| 1977 | Carina | F | Maiden | Greek | 235 |
| 1978 | Coen | M | | | 235 |
| 1979 | Jasmin | F | Fragrant flower | Arabic | 235 |
| 1980 | Jaylin | F | | | 235 |
| 1981 | Leighton | M | From the meadow farm | Old English | 235 |
| 1982 | Margo | F | Pearl | French | 235 |
| 1983 | Mustafa | M | | | 235 |
| 1984 | Reuben | M | Behold a son | Hebrew | 235 |
| 1985 | Arlette | F | Pledge | Old English | 234 |
| 1986 | Blaise | M | Stammered | Latin | 234 |
| 1987 | Dimitri | M | Of the earth | Greek | 234 |
| 1988 | Ayan | M | | | 234 |
| 1989 | Queen | F | | | 234 |
| 1990 | Robyn | F | | | 234 |
| 1991 | Valery | F | | | 234 |
| 1992 | Jenesis | F | | | 233 |
| 1993 | Keenan | M | Ancient | Irish | 233 |

| | | | | | |
|---|---|---|---|---|---|
| 1994 | Van | M | | | 233 |
| 1995 | Achilles | M | | | 232 |
| 1996 | Anniston | F | | | 232 |
| 1997 | Devyn | F | Poet | Irish | 232 |
| 1998 | Elia | F | The Lord is my God | Hebrew | 232 |
| 1999 | Lilia | F | | | 232 |
| 2000 | Aislinn | F | Vision | Irish | 231 |

The meaning of these names is only to orientate the reader. The top right column is the number of baby born in 2017 that have that name, ordered from more popular to less one.

## I still want more names!!!!

You can download or search the full list of names from the US Census Bureau website.

https://www.ssa.gov/oact/babynames/

# BABY NAMES WORKSHEET

Select the names that you like. Then place a tick next to the names that you like best.

| # | Name | Origin | Meaning | Like |
|---|------|--------|---------|------|
| 1 | | | | |
| 2 | | | | |
| 3 | | | | |
| 4 | | | | |
| 5 | | | | |
| 6 | | | | |
| 7 | | | | |
| 8 | | | | |
| 9 | | | | |
| 10 | | | | |
| 11 | | | | |
| 12 | | | | |
| 13 | | | | |
| 14 | | | | |
| 15 | | | | |
| 16 | | | | |
| 17 | | | | |
| 18 | | | | |
| 19 | | | | |
| 20 | | | | |
| 21 | | | | |
| 22 | | | | |
| 23 | | | | |
| 24 | | | | |
| 25 | | | | |
| 26 | | | | |
| 27 | | | | |
| 28 | | | | |
| 29 | | | | |
| 30 | | | | |

# ABOUT THE AUTHOR

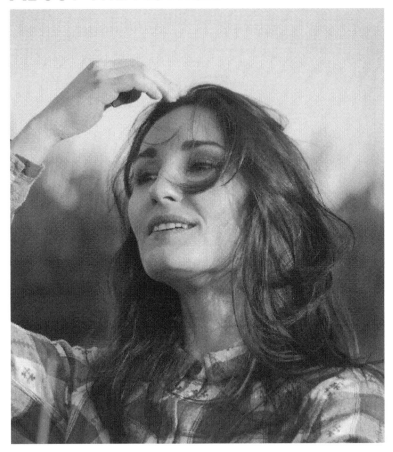

AUTHOR NAME is RUSTY COVE-SMITH

Find out more at amazon.com author page

Or visit https://gimbooks.info/team/rusty-cove-smith/